Praise and Recommendations
for *Live Calm with Cancer (and Beyond...)*

"This book is a MUST-READ by anyone whose life has been touched by a major illness like cancer! The authors take you into their private lives in a totally engaging way and provide invaluable tools to deal with all of the stress you are facing right now. Whether you are the one who is diagnosed or a care-giver, this book provides what you need. You will find comfort and the most powerful tools available to help you transcend the challenges you are facing right now and hasten your healing on all levels!"
—Diana Kirschner, PhD, bestselling author of *The Diamond Self Secret*

"Facing cancer is one of life's most difficult challenges. From long clinical experience, I know the value of staying centered and cultivating appreciation and forgiveness when dealing with this disease. Based on the author's personal experience and a clear understanding of the issues, *Live Calm With Cancer* skillfully guides the reader through these choppy waters through rich and practical mindfulness tools. Even people that are not diagnosed with major medical illnesses will benefit from this book."
—Frederic Luskin, Ph.D. Lecturer Stanford University School of Medicine and Author *Forgive for Good* and *Stress Free for Good*

"A cancer diagnosis can be a devastating blow. At the same time, it can also be a courageous and beautiful opportunity for discovering inner depth. Authors Tamara Green and David Dachinger have written *Live Calm with Cancer*, a precious and sacred guide. This book is for anyone whose life has been touched by cancer and you're open to the possibility of embracing its gifts of love and forgiveness."
—Dr. Shawne Duperon, Project Forgive Founder, 2016 Nobel Peace Prize Nominee

"A heart-felt, wise, honest, and tender book. Enormously helpful to those facing cancer, to the medical establishment, and to their loved ones. With easy, mindful tips and visceral meditations, authors David and Tamara take the reader on a journey through their Stage IV cancer experience, to the other side, to mentor readers on how to be calm and grounded even through challenging days! *Live Calm with Cancer (and Beyond)* is highly recommended -- this page turner is a cellular sensation!"
—Debbi Dachinger, bestselling author, media personality

"A deeply moving and profound book! *Live Calm With Cancer (and Beyond...)* shows how, with courage and determination, those living with cancer can overcome big challenges and get back to thriving. This inspiring journey of discovery illustrates how mindfulness can transform lives and empowers us all."
—Teresa de Grosbois, #1 International bestselling author of *Mass Influence - the Habits of the Highly Influential*

"At a critical time, when your world stops, this wonderful book *"Live Calm With Cancer (and Beyond...)"* will guide you through your medical circumstances with calm and ease. With wisdom and compassion, the authors of this critically important work have filled it with quick yet powerful mindfulness tips and soul-reaching meditations. If you've been feeling overwhelmed by the challenges of serious illness, this book has the keys to unlocking the answers."
—Partha Nandi, MD, FACP, Practicing Physician, Host and Creator, *Ask Dr Nandi*, Emmy award winning television show and International Best Selling Author, *Ask Dr Nandi: 5 Steps to Becoming Your Own #HealthHero for Longevity, Well-Being, and a Joyful Life*

"People with life-threatening illnesses are understandably stressed and overwhelmed. Tamara Green and David Dachinger bring their personal experience in overcoming cancer to inspire those that are facing all types of dangerous situations. They provide practical tools for managing the floods of emotion associated with critical illness. I highly recommend this book, which helps both patients and their caring family members, to navigate medical treatment with much more ease and calm."
—Steven M Kubersky MD

"I wish I had this book when my family was going through cancer! What a difference it could've made! The authors, a stage IV cancer patient and his caregiver, generously share the mindful tips they used to get through their medical ordeal. Not only do I highly recommend this book, but I also strongly encourage you to get their LovingMeditations app. The programs, which are specifically designed for those going through cancer and other major illnesses, will inspire you, give you hope and help you through your most difficult days."
—Viki Winterton, Founder and CEO, Expert Insights Publishing

Live Calm
With
Cancer
(and Beyond…)

TAMARA GREEN, LCSW

and DAVID DACHINGER

Mind Health, LLC
Mamaroneck, NY 10543

Cover Images:
macrovector © 123RF.com
wavebreakmediamicro © 123RF. com

DEDICATION

This book is dedicated to the millions of courageous and resolute souls worldwide who are living with cancer… and beyond.

CONTENTS

ACKNOWLEDGMENTS

We are eternally grateful for the boundless, unwavering support of all the people and organizations that inspired us to document our cancer journey. Living life while navigating major illness and co-authoring this book have been labors of love, and transformed us to the core.

Thank you...

- For the continuous support of our wonderful Evolutionary Business Council friends and colleagues, who initially inspired us to chronicle our story. You are the best!

- To David's rock-steady brothers of IAFF Local 1739, especially Rick, Dave, Tony, Guy, Tim, John and Rommie, and to our firehouse dispatchers.

- To the talented and dedicated doctors, nurses, and staff of WestMed Group, White Plains Hospital (especially Kristine and Clarissa), Beth Israel Medical Center, and NYU Langone Medical Center.

- To Dr. Dain Heer for the generosity of your time, brilliant teachings and powerful guidance.

- To Dan and Mitch of Crusoe Ventures for your immense contribution to the design of our beautiful *Loving Meditations* app.

- For our amazing friends who showed up for us during treatment, kept us fed, shoveled our driveway, and cheered us on every step of the way. We couldn't have gotten it done without you: Diane, Bettina & David, Larry & Andrea, Steve & Debbie, Jon & Marj, Steve & Amy, and Radical Rob.

- To Tamara's generous book club gang who made and delivered home cooked meals to our door every week. Soraya, Nancy, and Margarita, we appreciate you so much!

- For years of constant validation, ardent support and wise mentoring, Drs. Diana and Sam Kirschner, we deeply value your generous nature and loving guidance.

- To Westchester Restorative Dentistry and Implantology, for your world-class compassion and care.

- To our dear friends Kristen, Tom, Christine B. and Debbie Z. for your daily prayers and supportive phone calls. Kristen, even while your beloved mother was dying of pancreatic cancer, you were there for us 100%!

- To our wonderful parents Ralph & Verna, Nadia, Carroll & Leonard, and Marianne & Carroll, for raising us to be the resilient and unique adults that we've become.

- To our loving, devoted and dedicated siblings, Debbi, Tim, Dennis, Denise, Garrick, and Andrew, for your endless care, compassion and moral support. We love you dearly.

- For our shining star, Sarah, the most beautiful daughter we could ever dream of. You're a computer whiz who devoted many hours to the initial design and ideas for our *Loving Meditations* app. We are deeply touched and so very proud of you!

- To the champion in our life, Mark. While braving your own illness you still gifted us with a steady supply of bear hugs, cheerful humor and uplifting attitude. We adore you!

- To my beloved, David: Every single day that I spend being your wife, I realize how fortunate I am to be living such an abundant and fulfilled life. You are the anchor that holds me in place and the sails, which take me on our beautiful journey called *marriage*. Even after four decades of knowing you: your iron determination and resilience astonish me; your music and talents astound me; and, your friendship and love deeply move me. My love for you has grown immensely with each blissful year of our union.

- To my earth-angel, Tamara: I'll never adequately express the gratitude, love and admiration I have for you. You are light and love personified. We've been on a fantastic life odyssey together!

You always bring out the absolute best in me (and everyone else). Sharing our cancer journey has brought us to an even deeper level of connection and compassion. I am humbled to be your friend and life-partner.

DISCLAIMER

This book contains the ideas and opinions of its authors. Please use common sense when using any meditation tools. For safety reasons, don't watch, listen to or use them while driving, operating any machinery or doing any activity requiring particular attention. This book is distributed with the understanding that the authors and publisher are not engaged in offering medical advice, diagnosis, treatment or any other kind of personal professional services in any manner.

Always seek the advice of your physician or any other qualified health provider with any questions you may have regarding any medical condition.

The authors and publisher specifically disclaim all responsibility for any injury, liability, loss or risk, personal or otherwise, which is incurred as a consequence, directly or indirectly, that may result from your use and application of any of the contents of this book.

CHAPTER 1
INTRODUCTION: LAUNCHING YOUR CALM

What's going on? How did this happen? What do I do? My life has turned completely upside down because of a stupid little six-letter word: CANCER! Help!

Cancer is life-altering. When newly diagnosed, it's overwhelming for the patient and care-partner. It's difficult to figure out what to do first! The doctors direct you or your loved one to the appropriate medical treatment. You numbly follow the instructions laid out before you, but inside, you're screaming.

It can take you down a dismal path, devastating the body, mind, and soul of everyone involved. It will have an impact on your physical comfort and your psychological and spiritual well-being.

According to the American Cancer Society, nearly one out of four cancer patients will be diagnosed with clinical depression at some point during the course of their illness. However, according to Cancer Research UK, maintaining a regular meditation practice has benefits such as relaxation, calm, peace of mind, clarity and insight, "which may improve your wellbeing and health."[1]

---

[1] "Meditation," Cancer Research UK, last modified February 5, 2015, accessed August 21, 2017, http://www.cancerresearchuk.org/about-cancer/cancer-in-general/treatment/complementary-alternative-

Care-partners experience their own difficulties. The American Cancer Society National Quality of Life Survey for Caregivers initiated an eight-year study in 2002.[2] Their findings show that depression, fear, anxiety, feeling overwhelmed, and even guilt are very common symptoms for the parents, spouses, and adult children who care for their loved ones with cancer.

But we have some heartening news: to date, there are over 163 studies that have shown that meditation and mindfulness techniques can reduce anxiety and stress, and might also help control problems such as pain, difficulty sleeping, tiredness, feeling sick, and high blood pressure.

Cancer did not conquer us and the main reason was our daily practice of meditation and mindfulness!

Our mission in writing this book is to bring calm and ease to what you're going through. In fact, we plan on giving you the kind of hope and optimism that will turn your cancer experience into a journey of self-discovery and recovery, like it did for us.

---

therapies/individual-therapies/meditation.

[2] Elizabeth Mendes, "Seven Key Findings From 8-Year Study of Cancer Caregivers," American Cancer Society, November 27, 2013, https://www.cancer.org/latest-news/seven-key-findings-from-8-year-study-of-cancer-caregivers.html.

Yes, cancer is a game-changer. But as you will find out in this book, it cannot conquer you—not if you let it. In fact, you can use the cancer experience to help you discover:

- How deeply you can love and be loved
- The tremendous power of hope and faith
- The ability to reach peace in the most excruciating moments
- How your confidence will most likely grow
- Who your true friends are
- How to release old painful memories and make wonderful new ones
- How courageous and strong you really are
- How your Spirit can awaken

As I (Tamara) prepare to write this book with my beloved, my heart is filled with gratitude. Early this morning, when David was leaving for his twenty-four-hour shift at the firehouse, he said with such tenderness, "I love you, honey." Then, during breakfast, our teenage son, Mark, and I laughed hysterically while playing cards (our daily routine for years). And, our college-aged daughter, Sarah, texted me to say, "Hi Mom, just thinking of you. Have a nice day." Wow! It's only 9:00 a.m. and I feel so fortunate to have such a loving, fun, and supportive family. I have an amazing extended family, friends, and clients, as well. Nowadays, I feel so fortunate to have these pinch-me kind of moments almost every day.

As you'll read in Chapter 2, however, my life wasn't all sunshine and roses. I did not feel gratitude, nor did I have a life that reflected anything to be grateful for. In fact, I spent much of my time in confusion, self-loathing, and even despair. In my past, I never could've imagined a life so wonderful. If someone would've predicted that I'd be so loved and admired, my insecure self would've said, "Stop telling lies! That can't be possible!" Yet, here I am, happy to be me and living a life that I love.

David, too, had his allotment of hardships throughout his life. Yet, for the purpose of this book, we will be sharing mostly about our biggest challenge thus far—our cancer journey.

David will impart his perspectives as a patient diagnosed with stage IV cancer. By the way, there is no *stage V* cancer. *Stage IV* means the cancer has spread from where it started to another organ or area of the body. In other words, it's as bad as cancer gets. In David's case, it had spread to the lymph nodes in his neck.

Throughout the book, David will reveal the challenges of being a cancer patient, from diagnosis to survivorship. Ah, *survivorship*, that's a wonderful word! Yes, David made it!

As his caregiver, you'll be hearing from me, too. I was right there by his side going through the pain, fear, and upset right along with him. I'll share how this experience moved me in ways I never expected, and how I found out who I really am—a woman who loves deeply and thoroughly, and a wife who will drop everything to be by her husband's side when he needs her the most.

Throughout each chapter, we share the mindfulness tools we used that helped us tremendously throughout our cancer adventure. These techniques even brought us closer together as a couple, helping us reach a higher level of love and understanding that we never dreamed possible.

Our desire is to make your life easier by guiding you through your most challenging moments. We will reveal the secrets to not only surviving, but also thriving as patient, caregiver, and survivor.

Navigating each challenge of our cancer voyage, we recognized that, as a result, we became more resilient, wise, and calm. It was as if we started out as navy seaman recruits and ended up fleet admirals. We marvel at how the most arduous moments turned into our biggest victories. It is through this excursion called cancer that we have found, once again, our commitment to one another and to life. We'd like this to happen for you, too.

Whether you are a patient, survivor or care-partner, the sole purpose of this book is to help you to become an active participant in your healing journey.

There are three ways to get the most out of this book:

1. Patient's perspective:

If you've ever been diagnosed with cancer, David certainly knows what you're going through. When you read his entries, you'll immediately get a sense of not being alone in this scary process. He writes about the experiences he had and the tools he used to get through them. Therefore, if you desire to jumpstart your healing journey, by all means read his input only, at least for now. Please do not skip the most important parts, however, which are the mindfulness tips and meditations contained in this book.

2. Caregiver's perspective:

If you are a care-partner, Tamara knows how you feel. In each chapter, she shares her perspectives, mindfulness tools, and meditation techniques that dramatically helped her through the sometimes-exhausting journey of caring for her loved ones.

3.   Shared perspective:

If you're a patient or survivor and would like to understand what it's like to stand in the shoes of your care-partner, or, vice versa, then please read both David and Tamara's entries. Doing so will broaden your understanding, compassion, and perspective for the entire experience.

Note: Keep in mind that even though this book is written as if we're speaking directly to those going through cancer, it can also be extremely helpful and powerful for anyone experiencing other major illnesses.

You'll benefit from reading this book if:

- you or your loved one has been diagnosed with cancer;
- you desire to actively participate in your healing journey;
- you are the caregiver to someone diagnosed with cancer;
- you are a survivor of cancer and are anxious about relapse;
- you experience anxiety and stress before or during each exam, procedure, test, or scan;

- you know someone who is living with cancer as either patient or caregiver, and you have a desire to be more helpful and to better understand his or her journey.

The fact that you're reading this book means you are ready to make significant changes for the better.

Chapters reflect each phase of our own cancer adventure. However, this may not be the exact experience you're having or in the same order:

- Before Cancer
- Diagnosis
- Treatment
- Surgery
- Survivorship

Less Stress and More Ease

Throughout the book we've included mindfulness tips, and a written guided meditation at the end of most chapters. However, you'll have a deeper experience by listening to each meditation on our app called *Loving Meditations* (available at www.calmcancerstress.com). The combination of Tamara's soothing guided voice, David's soul-moving music, and stunning imagery are quite impactful. Here's a rave by one of our app users:

> This app, *Loving Meditations*, is beyond fabulous. I've had it for several months and use it daily, often several times a day. There are specific meditations for cancer patients and their caregivers, but many are powerful meditations for anyone. Some are very short that easily lifts your mood. Others are longer that help you remain calm and peaceful during chemo, pain, worry and anxiety. Others are powerful aids for sleep, appreciating the positives, and attracting what you desire, such as, healing, peace, or comfort. I listen to the *Awaken Allow and Attract* meditation every day and I swear it's helping me to be more financially successful in my business! Tamara's voice is clear, beautiful, and uplifting, the background music is wonderful and the mesmerizing images add a whole new element of beauty and calm. I've been recommending this app to people who have any health problems (not just cancer), to those in good health who desire a meditation practice, or, for those who want to strengthen the meditation routine they already have. For beginners, there's even a short guide on how to meditate successfully. —Judith Joshel, Love and Relationship Coach

The definition of *mindfulness* in *Merriam-Webster* is "the practice of maintaining a nonjudgmental state of heightened or complete awareness of one's thoughts, emotions, or experiences on a moment-to-moment basis."[3]

You'll be delighted to know that you have mindful moments all the time. For example, have you noticed how completely relaxed and present you are when deeply engrossed in a book, movie, or hobby? That, my friend, is mindfulness.

For example, Tamara has a new passion for coloring, because she finds it relaxing and enjoyable. Dr. Stan Rodski, a peak-performance neuroscientist, created a coloring book for adults called *Anti-stress: Meditation Through Coloring*. Tamara found that by focusing on the task of coloring, she shifted from feeling pressured and stressed (BETA brainwave state) to feeling very relaxed (ALPHA brainwave state). Ahhh, being in the ALPHA state feels so good.

Go ahead and see how quick and easy it is to become calm, present, and in the state of ALPHA by trying the mindfulness tip below.

---

[3] *Merriam-Webster Unabridged Dictionary*, s.v. "mindfulness," accessed August 21, 2017, http://unabridged.merriam-webster.com/unabridged/mindfulness.

Mindful Tip

Sit comfortably and lower your shoulders. Breathe in through your nose and focus on the sensation of bringing fresh air into your lungs and expanding your chest. Hold the breath for one second and notice the internal vibration at the top of this breath. Then exhale through your mouth and notice the sensation of air leaving your lungs. Repeat five to ten times, or until you feel completely relaxed and focused on your body.

History of Meditation

For thousands of years, different forms of meditation have been spread by Taoist China, Buddhist India, the Bhagavad Gita and yoga masters such as Patanjali. Meditation has expanded throughout the world and is widely known for its benefits. The type of meditation offered in this book is not the kind where we have you sit in a lotus position for hours, with thumbs and middle fingers touching, eyes closed. Instead, we offer mindfulness-based stress reduction (MBSR), or guided, meditation.

Since the late 1970's, meditation has become increasingly more common and popular. Today, wellness programs that include mindful programs are ubiquitous in settings like hospitals, the work place, senior living facilities, and even on Capitol Hill. It is now estimated that one in seven Americans has meditated. Many highly visible athletes, musicians, actors and executives have mindful practices which help them manage their stress and improve their performance.

Benefits of Meditation:

Meditation reduces stress. Research shows that a regular practice of calming the mind, even minutes per day, reduces the stress hormone cortisol, leaving you feeling more peaceful and grounded.

Meditation generates presence. Because most thinking is judgment-based, *if you're thinkin', you're stinkin'*. For example, when you're fixated on your past, you're probably feeling regret, anger, or upset. When you're engrossed in thoughts of your future, you're probably feeling anxious or worried. *Presence* occurs when your mind is neutral (no judgment). Even thirty seconds of meditation or mindfulness can create presence and ease.

Meditation helps tune you into your inner guidance. Tai Chi master Ilchee Lee said, "Where your mind goes, energy goes." That's true! And, what you focus on expands. There are three major energy centers in your body, located at the forehead (third eye chakra), chest (heart chakra), and lower belly (sacral chakra). When the energy is balanced among all three centers, you feel at peace and grounded, regardless of your situation or circumstances. Most people spend way too much time thinking, which produces a congestion of energy in the mind. This then initiates an energy imbalance, leading to stress. Because it facilitates presence, meditation helps to lower and equalize the energy from your head (center for creativity) into your heart (inner wisdom) and lower belly (gut intuition), establishing harmony among all three energy centers. This, in turn, tunes you into pure awareness and the realm of possibilities.

Meditation facilitates receiving. There's nothing in this world that's not energy. At any particular time, you're either giving, receiving, blocking, or playing with (manipulating) energy. Receiving energy is actually very difficult for many people. When you have a problem, notice how you're blocking or not receiving energy. For example, a love problem is a receiving-love problem and a money problem is a receiving-money problem. Meditation enables you to be in the space of receiving and allowing. Because the Universe continuously desires to give to you, a practice of meditation is synonymous with receiving a daily dose of unconditional love. How does it get better than that?

Meditation sharpens the mind. A relaxed mind enhances focus and creativity. For example, 95 percent of our writing creativity is a direct result of going within and listening. A breathing meditation oxygenates the brain, leaving you feeling revitalized and refreshed within minutes. For an immediate result, try the mindfulness tip above—with sharp inhales and audible exhales. Keep repeating this breathing technique until you feel refreshed and revitalized. Enjoy the increased ability to concentrate and be laser focused.

Meditation stabilizes emotions. Studies show that a daily meditation practice can protect you from depression, stress, and anxiety. This is true for teens as well as adults.

Meditation regulates the healing journey. Along with exercise, meditation has huge benefits to the physical body. One study showed that employees who had a regular practice of quiet contemplation missed less work than those who did not.

Meditation helps you actualize your goals. This certainly has been true for many of Tamara's clients. She finds that the ones who commit to a daily practice of going within are ten times more likely to see their dreams come true. Very exciting!

With such a great list of benefits for meditation, how could you go wrong? No more excuses, okay? Happy Meditating!

CHAPTER 2
REWIND: LIFE BEFORE CANCER

David

My freshman year, college was not going well. As an aeronautical engineering major at a Big Ten university, I was struggling with the curriculum and receiving lousy grades. A native New Yorker, I was culture-shocked living in a midwestern railroad town, and my roommate loathed me. I suffered brutal sore throats and the flu on a regular basis. I felt out of my element. Unhappy and depressed, I was living in a no-choice universe, convinced that I had to pursue a path completely asynchronous with my soul's purpose. I didn't realize there was any other choice until a friend said, "You're obviously not happy here. You absolutely love music, so why don't you pursue that?"

What a gift this was! I'd been more concerned with pleasing my father by following in his footsteps in the airline industry than with following my true passion. Once I recognized that my friend's advice was a lifeboat the universe was sending to save me from this gloomy existence, I took action and transferred. This was an incredible liberation, a chance to reinvent myself and pursue the right career. Once I transitioned to music school in Boston, my reality became lighter, happier, and more fulfilling.

I like to believe everything always works out for me. I've often repeated it like a mantra. And I often remind myself: I've been blessed with a good life.

While I recognize I've been blessed, some blessings are not immediately obvious. What may appear to be a painful, difficult life situation can be a gift in disguise. On occasion, it's taken years to appreciate what the actual benefit is. My life's been touched by good fortune and numerous adversities. In an effort to make sense of one of my biggest challenges, I've recorded the story of what happened before, during, and after cancer.

As for the obvious gifts, the life I've lived looks pretty good, with a wonderful wife and terrific kids. I work (actually it's more like play) in two dream careers. Today I'm composing music for the NFL, PGA, or NCAA; tomorrow I'll be responding to emergencies on a crimson fire engine. My work/play jobs afford me the platform to reach millions with my music, and the opportunity to be of service to the public as a firefighter and Advanced Emergency Medical Technician (AEMT).

I've written music that's been heard by over 1.5 billion people during network TV broadcasts of events like the Super Bowl; the Masters, one of professional golf's most prestigious tournaments; and NCAA March Madness. My compositions have underscored the epic moments of athletes like Tiger Woods, Arnold Palmer, Tom Brady, and Peyton Manning. As a fan, I've always loved the excitement and drama of sports, particularly when monumental achievements unfold. In TV sports, key highlights of the events are edited together like a movie trailer, and my music serves to enhance the spectacle and excitement. Or it can add an emotional underscore to a poignant, heartwarming story. By heightening the viewer's experience, the music I create functions like a movie soundtrack.

I've noticed that a pattern emerges when I create these soundtracks. It's a steady formula, but also supports spontaneity. There are two elements: constancy and allowance. In other words, be consistent in the practice and be open to allowing what is possible. This blueprint works for me as a composer, but also applies to facing life challenges like major illness. It eases the journey.

Most of the music I write starts with a foundation, typically a drumbeat or chord pattern. In real life, this equates to having a consistent, daily practice of nurturing body and soul—baseline actions like regular exercise and eating healthy foods. Meditation, yoga, positive thinking, and mindfulness also contribute to maintaining that solid foundation, returning benefits of mental and physical resilience, both daily, and during tough times like coping with cancer.

The next step in my music creation process is to build on this foundation by adding different instruments. In virtually all of my musical productions, less is more. By following this minimalist approach, there's space for sonic events to exist without clutter and distraction. There's less competition between each element. Often, it's a challenge to write so minimally. I have to resist my natural tendency to pile on more layers, which can result in a complex and muddy wall of sound.

The solution is to simplify: pare down the density and complexity. Practically every time I allow more space to exist, the music breathes and feels better. I've found this can also apply to life situations. For example, in my cancer journey, when I put some space around the judgments and conclusions I made about my cancer diagnosis and treatment, I stopped seeing having cancer as a tragic event or failure. I shifted my point of view away from *this is something really bad happening to me*. Instead, I invited the space of allowance, grace, and gratitude to my daily experience. Fresh outlooks on living with cancer emerged. I'd ask myself, "What other perspective is possible? Is there something positive to be found in all this?"

Over a career of writing music, I've found it really helps to let go of attachment to the song and the outcome of the process. Like a living thing, the song becomes its own entity, and will show me where it needs to go. Resist this direction, and the results tend to be mediocre. When I release attachment to how I've decided the piece should evolve, the music is more authentic and accessible.

In my cancer experience, simply not judging the process was highly effective. By going with the flow and being at one with *what is*, I found less persistence of pain and anxiety.

When I don't immediately conclude something is good or bad, I can view it just as it is: the new song I created (as opposed to "my latest bomb"). Then, if I choose, I can move beyond to something else. Often a greater possibility is just around the corner. The initial composition (or life experience) may simply be a necessary stepping-stone on the path to a better, happier result. In contrast, judging that something is wrong is to presume to know the full trajectory that life (or music) will follow.

There's a saying: Don't quit five minutes before the miracle happens. We may think we know what's supposed to be happening right now and where it's all leading. How can we be so sure when we're only seeing a few pixels of the big picture? Could something unexpectedly wonderful happen when we keep faith and stay the course?

Amazingly, Abraham Lincoln's path to the White House included eight election defeats, two businesses failures, and a nervous breakdown. Yet Lincoln is regarded as one of America's greatest presidents, and he overcame the failures that initially blocked his route. Lincoln didn't judge these defeats enough to prevent him from persisting and achieving greatness.

Great musicians talk about being a vessel for the music. They speak about getting out of the way and allowing the magic to happen. Clearly there's a greater wisdom available if we understand how to tap into it. What typically blocks the flow of this universal intelligence is our actively chattering minds. Our non-stop thoughts easily distract us from receiving this higher level of guidance and instinct. We must somehow quiet the mental noise and tune into the special assistance that's available.

As a composer, I've never really experienced writer's block. I go in the studio every day, and without expectation, I simply write. I sketch ideas with my Pro Tools software like a curious gardener planting a variety of seeds. With the proper care, some will blossom into beautiful flowers, some will turn out to be weeds. My practice of writing without expectation is liberating, because the judgment of outcome is removed. Similarly, I approached living with cancer by letting go of my attachment to outcome. Not forming conclusions about events, meanings, and circumstances opened the door for other possibilities to exist.

Some of the most incredible musical moments I've had were when I made a so-called "mistake." While writing music for the PGA Championship, I had recorded a violin and bagpipes for a Scottish effect to echo the links-style golf course at Whistling

Straits. When I cut and pasted the violin's audio, I accidentally placed it off the beat. At that very moment, I created something completely different from what I had intended. For that split second, I got out of the way. At first, I judged it as sounding wrong. Then I recognized the brilliance of this gift, because it was far more interesting than anything I would've consciously or deliberately written. I embraced the mistake—suddenly the best musical moment of this important show-opener.

Having cancer may seem like wrongness, a mistake in our grand plan of life. Certainly, it was a totally different reality than what I had in mind. But what if cancer is also a gift? Perhaps it's an opportunity to press the reset switch, reinvent ourselves, grow, embrace humility, and learn self-compassion. What if cancer entering our world can lead us to a life of increased gratitude and appreciation?

Long before cancer became a personal reality, I had much to be grateful for. But in my first four decades I really "efforted" to get what I desired, and often struggled without success. For example, my search for a life partner was a long and painful process. I did not invite what is possible. Instead I focused on what's not possible.

When Tamara and I met during her freshman year of college, I didn't believe it was conceivable that this amazing woman and I could be friends, let alone enjoy a long-term relationship. I saw only the obvious limitations preventing it—me living in Boston, her in L.A., me not feeling worthy of dating such a beautiful woman—so I couldn't even picture how our lives could ever align. I easily judged and concluded that these things clearly weren't going to happen. This contributed to a very lengthy off-and-on relationship that wouldn't totally solidify for seventeen years.

In hindsight, I guess I needed to get all those years of doubting and judging out of the way. Once free of such mental roadblocks, I could actualize and help start creating the life we share today.

I had always been thankful for lifelong good health, but nowhere near as much as I was after the cancer diagnosis. I appreciated Tamara's love and care, but that experience was profoundly changed by our caregiver–patient relationship. I was grateful for my freedom to do anything I desired, including working as a firefighter and competing as an athlete. But that feeling turned into an aching grief when I had to stop working, and felt too weak to go to the gym. I valued my friends, family, and coworkers before cancer entered the picture; however, my relationships transformed dramatically with many of them during the cancer journey.

Cancer had touched my life a few times. I witnessed my grandfather, a prolific inventor, author, and teacher, wind down his life during his retirement in Florida. Always ahead of his time with health and nutrition, he was charismatic and popular. I derived my love of sports and music from him, and in many ways he was a father to me.

In his later years, I sensed that my grandfather made a pivotal decision while living in a senior community. He seemed to stop taking care of himself. In 1983, when he was diagnosed with colon cancer, I visited him several times during his last months. The reality of actually knowing someone with cancer was a strange new personal episode. It seemed he was spiraling down to a place where no one could help him. Perhaps he was preparing to check out. As he faded mentally and physically, I had my first experience of someone close to me dying, and it left a profound and lasting mark.

I considered the meaning of his leaving the earth that way. Did he make a conscious or unconscious decision to pass on? What had changed for him? How could someone who was so vital and health-conscious his whole life get so sick? Was it selfish for me to expect him to keep living if he was ready to transition?

I was also absorbing a lot of information about his medical care and the hospital. I concluded that the HMO in Florida was offering shoddy care, the doctors didn't give a crap, and no one was really trying to help him. Family members stepped in as patient advocates to ensure the medical care was adequate, but I kept getting the impression that the system wasn't working to help my grandfather get well. This all burned a vivid perception in my mind of what cancer, oncological care, and dying looked like.

About fifteen years later, I had my second experience with someone I was close to being diagnosed with cancer. This was my good friend and music-business associate Mike, whom I'd known for thirty-plus years. Mike was diagnosed with a brain tumor, following which I visited him frequently in his Manhattan office. It was surreal to see Mike's sharp mental acuity gradually eroded by cancer. Much of his attention was focused on continuing his legacy when he was no longer on this earth. Again I decided, "So this is what cancer looks like." It seemed essentially invisible. Something was taking place inside Mike that was only noticeable because of his diminishing mental status. A malignant entity was growing inside Mike's brain, out of everyone's sight except his doctors'.

I felt profound loss when Mike succumbed to cancer, and again felt confused. How could this happen to someone who was always so healthy, positive, and loving?

As a kid I wasn't sick much, and when I did get typical childhood diseases like chickenpox, mumps, and measles, my mother would praise me about how mild my symptoms were compared to those of other children. This helped me form a self-image of, *I'm healthy with a good immune system.* I wasn't hospitalized except for the removal of my tonsils at age five, which was a very common procedure for kids in the 1960s.

As an adult, I developed a bit of cockiness about how healthy I was. My body was reliable, solid, never really getting ill, never letting me down. Perhaps I even felt a little superior to the patients I cared for as an advanced EMT who were the same general age as I was but who were dealing with major medical problems. My opportunity to be completely humbled was just around the corner, and it unfolded in a very peculiar way....

Mindful Tip to Calm the Emotions

Pause. Stop what you are doing. Acknowledge what you are feeling (anger, frustration, sadness, etc.). Labeling your feelings is the first step to calming your emotions. Take ten deep breaths. Getting oxygen into your system instantly begins the calming process.

TAMARA

1. Blue Eyes

At age five, I already had a strong sense of people and what made them tick. I knew the importance of love and kindness toward self and others. In fact, my doll, Heidi, was constantly the subject of my attention and affection. My fantasy was always her turning to me for help and guidance, pretending she was upset about some unkind thing said or done to her. As her devoted friend, my self-imposed job was to help her feel better by saying, "Heidi, don't you know how special you are? They just said those things because they're sad and taking it out on you. You are amazing!"

I would imagine that Heidi said, "Thanks Tammy, I feel better. Let's go tell them to play with us so they don't feel so sad anymore."

I spent hours in this kind of loving and supportive play with my inanimate yet intimate friend. In the let's-help-people-feel-better bubble that occupied hours of each day, I assumed everyone focused on such things. Little did I know that my role-play with Heidi was preparation for my profession as a psychotherapist some twenty-five years later.

Between the ages of eleven and seventeen, many changes occurred within me and my family—including raging adolescent hormones and my parents splitting and subsequent remarriages to new partners. Family events and holidays suddenly included new and instant grandparents, aunts, uncles, sisters, and brothers. Some were wonderful new additions I happily welcomed into my life, yet others, not so much. There were two men in particular who were lost and unhappy, often turning to for me for comfort and solace in very inappropriate ways. They sought me out, pulled me away from the others and took away my innocence.

During these troubling years, all I had known and trusted seemed to vanish into thin air. I longed for the return of my five-year-old innocent and confident Tammy. In my own dungeon of confusion, shame, and self-loathing, I locked myself away, convinced of being unworthy of love and believing I had to deal with this inner torment alone. One by one, I separated myself from my best friends and confidants. The happy child within seemed gone forever.

During my prison term in seclusion, taking the bus to school no longer seemed an option. Since we lived on almost three acres of avocado trees, I worked the orchard during the summers to make money. My plan was to acquire enough to buy myself a bicycle and ride to school—anything to steer clear of my friends who rode that bus. It took me three summers of wielding tall ladders, picking poles and heavy wooden boxes filled with the olive-green fruit to save enough for my new ten-speed bike.

What freedom I felt as I ventured my way from home to school and back again each day! A three-hour roundtrip commute within fourteen hilly miles became my daily retreat from suffering. Thank God, I had found a way to cope! I couldn't tell if it was the solitude or the sweat that created more bliss within me.

My teenage years weren't easy, but I sure learned to love all things athletic. I joined the track team and my delighted coach cheered as I won blue ribbons in the mile relay. My tough dance teacher honored me with a position in her modern dance program. Always looking for new adventures, I tried out for the volleyball, swim, and water polo teams. I started a backpacking club where we trekked the trails of the Sierra Nevada Mountain Range for three weeks at a time. Sports was not only my therapy, but also my sanctuary.

Besides athletics, becoming a Trojan at University of Southern California (USC) was just what my psyche needed. It was my fresh start. New friends, fun classes, and varsity crew were my tickets to salvation.

In my freshman year, I lived with my new roommate, Debbi. The moment we met, we became instant friends. A drama major with a big personality and tons of fun, Debbi was a transplant from New York. Just hearing her Long Island accent made me smile.

"Thank God it's Friday!" I exclaimed as I completed the last chapter of my reading assignment. Looking up from my book, I noticed that Debbi was not sitting at her usual spot on her twin bed in our closet-sized dorm room. I walked into the hallway to stretch my limbs, and something at the other end of the corridor caught my attention. This good-looking guy was walking into the hallway from the Common Room. He had dark hair and the bluest eyes I had ever seen. Within seconds, our gaze locked with serious electric energy happening between us. It felt like a *zap*! It was a wonderfully powerful feeling.

Who is this guy and where did he come from? I excitedly thought to myself. Suddenly, Debbi appeared behind him, entering from the Common Room, as well. Waving me over, she said, "Meet my brother, David. He's here for a couple of days from Boston. David, meet my roomie, Tamara." That's when he flashed his smile, leaving me weak in the knees. I was instantly enamored.

Over the course of his visit, Debbi and I showed Blue Eyes the expansive UCS campus, including the Rose Garden and LA Coliseum. The next day, we ventured off campus, visiting the Chinese Mann Theatre (now the Grauman's Chinese Theater) and the five-pointed brass stars embedded in the sidewalks of the

Hollywood Walk of Fame. On day three, I borrowed my friend's Volkswagen Beetle and we headed for Santa Monica State Beach. We roasted like marshmallows, returning burnt and blissfully happy. David and I, smitten and googly-eyed, were unable to leave each other's side. That night, we snuck away from Debbi to get some alone time. On the top floor of the USC parking garage, we spent the entire night talking, using the VW Bug as our shelter and getaway.

That night I learned that Blue Eyes also came from a broken home. After his parents' divorce, he became the man of the house way too young. He had wanted to become an airline pilot, in the same industry as his father, but ended up following his lifelong enthusiasm for music. He played the saxophone in a popular and steadily booked group called The Allston Funk Band. I found him to be smart and talented, yet humble and unassuming. From sundown to sunup, we talked easily and endlessly, still sharing our dreams while witnessing an orange and pink sunrise, which displayed a spectacular array of muted colors that only LA's smog could produce.

After only three days, I felt closer to Blue Eyes than anyone else in my life. Days later, I received his first of many letters (this was in 1977—way before email). He talked of visiting LA again during the summer months. I eagerly replied, encouraging his visit.

Summer came and we spent three glorious weeks together. We fell in love. Wishing to leave behind the cold winters of Boston, he shared his dream of living somewhere near the beach. We fantasized about being together forever and promised to stay in contact. However, youth and three thousand miles between us made it difficult to honor this pledge. We wouldn't see each other again for another four years.

With my unresolved childhood wounds plaguing me, at age twenty-three, I was hopelessly insecure and unhappy again. On the outside, however, everything looked and smelled like roses: a college graduate; an employee of a high-paying corporate job; friends; a social life; and a fair relationship with my family, including my stepparents. Yet, inside the roses were wilted and even rotting. I felt deeply lost and bitter.

One morning, feeling particularly low, I jumped into my 2-door silver Honda Civic hoping that I could drive away my dark thoughts. I headed for the San Gabriel Mountains, a place that usually lifted my spirits. However, the more I drove, the more alone and hopeless I felt. After reaching the mountain's peak at Angeles Crest Highway, I looped the car around, heading back down the very windy San Gabriel Canyon Road. Going way too fast through the steep turns, I reflected on all the years I had spent feeling shame, and how inner peace seemed unreachable.

Then, a thought crossed my mind: *Tamara, just let go of the steering wheel, crash through the guardrail, and fly over the cliff to certain death.* As the next hairpin turn approached, this deadly thought actually sounded good to me. I loosened my grip on the steering wheel, using only my index fingers to steer. Ready to say goodbye to this painful world, I counted down out loud, "Three... two... one...," closed my eyes and let go of the wheel, then suddenly screamed "NO!" at which point I grabbed the wheel again and slammed on my brakes. Shaking uncontrollably, I slowly maneuvered the car onto the shoulder to safety. And then, the torrent of tears was finally unleashed.

After thirteen years of pent-up misery, I wrapped my arms tightly around my belly and wailed. Wracked with emotional pain, I rocked back and forth in the driver's seat and cried for the death of my innocence. I cried for blaming myself all those years and for being unable to look into the mirror without hating myself. When I thought I was done crying, more waves of sorrow washed over me, requiring one tearful release after the other. I even cried for the men who made me feel this way, knowing that as perpetrators, their pain had to be much more brutal than mine.

During that hour of weepy surrender, the chains that held me to my past began to loosen. A tiny ripple of liberation surged through my veins. Although trembling and exhausted, something inside of me knew I was going to be okay.

The next day, I made my first appointment with a therapist. It was the first time I heard the words *sexual molestation,* a new term in the '80s. *Wow! They actually had a label that described what happened to me,* I thought. My counselor assured me that it was not my fault, that I wasn't to blame, and that the feeling of shame was not only normal but also common. I remember sitting in her office thinking, *Maybe I'm not such a terrible person after all?* It was a revelation, an epiphany that launched my lifelong journey of self-discovery, or rediscovery.

A couple of months after my twenty-sixth birthday, Debbi called to announce that her brother was in LA. Apparently, Blue Eyes had expressed a wish to see me. I welcomed the invitation to meet for dinner with Debbi, David, and their mother. As I entered the restaurant, he walked up to greet me and that wonderful electric energy between us was still there. *Zap! Zing!*

After the meal, walking me to my car, he asked to see me again the following day. We agree to meet at a local Mexican joint in Long Beach near my apartment. By the end of this meal, we talked of love and a desire to commit to one another. After eight years, we were finally a couple.

Our long-distance relationship between New York and California consisted of phone calls, letters, and tape recordings. As a result, we connected nearly every day. Eighteen months later, Blue Eyes fulfilled his dream of living in Southern California as we moved into our new one-bedroom apartment only one block from the beach. Within six months, we were engaged to be married.

As a recording engineer, David's talents were in demand and kept him commuting to New York and New Jersey, mixing one album after the next. The constant travel proved difficult, so we decided to move to New York together. Having no passion at all for my corporate job, I happily agreed to leave LA County, my home since birth, to experience the Big Apple. However, money was tight and we could only afford an apartment in Hoboken, New Jersey.

With moving day only three months away, I found myself becoming increasingly nervous when he talked of our future marriage. Even though we got along great, I became progressively anxious. My thoughts, which I should've shared with David, were: *I wish we could slow everything down; marriage scares me; I'm going to screw everything up; I know we'll end up divorced, just like our parents.* Three weeks before moving day, I broke off our engagement.

Heartbroken, David left again for the East and I remained in the West. Once again, I felt utterly lost.

The next eight years proved to be the most important undertaking of my life: my self-exploration. With therapy, yoga, and meditation as my primary focus, I truly found myself. It was a slow yet worthwhile ride of turning my wrongness into my strongness.

Recalling my excitement about living on the East Coast, I sold all of my belongings, making a total of $700. With it, I purchased a one-way ticket on United and paid for a two week stay in a low-budget motel. With $36 in my pocket, and ready for my life to take flight in a new direction, I headed to my new home— New York City.

With a strong desire to become a psychotherapist, I got my master's degree in social work at Fordham University, did post-graduate training for couples and family therapy at the Ackerman Institute for the Family, and worked full-time in state and private hospitals as a psychiatric social worker. Tammy's let's-help-people-feel-better bubble came alive once again! In the early 1990s, I hung my psychotherapy shingle outside of my office, announcing to the world that my dream had come true.

By the age of 36, I had dated a lot of men, but never forgot about Blue Eyes. It had been eight years since I had seen or talked to him. Even though I had wonderful memories of our relationship, I rejected my urges to contact him. Plain and simple, I was too scared, and was determined to find someone else who gave me a similar electrical connection, but no one else came close.

And then, on a sunny yet chilly day in late February, there he was. Blue Eyes was walking his dog down West Seventy-Fourth Street. *ZAP!* The electricity was still there for me! I was ecstatic to see him, waved and said "Hi!" But he was not smiling. In fact, he gave me a death stare and walked right past me, leaving me trembling with regret on that brownstone-lined street in Manhattan.

Two weeks went by and I couldn't stop thinking about him and what a tragedy it was that we were not on speaking terms. Because our relationship had ended so painfully, I couldn't blame him. Determined to do whatever it took to make amends, I searched and found his number in the phone book (pre-internet), and drummed up the courage to call. I dialed, got his answering machine, and spoke nervously, "Hi David, this is Tamara. I'd like to make amends to you. I'll do whatever it takes for us to be at least friendly. Please call me ... but I'll understand if you don't."

A very long three weeks later, he called back and said with a chill in his voice, "I'll hear you out." We made arrangements to meet on a Sunday. We talked for four hours while walking through Central Park. We met several more times hashing things out, answering long overdue questions and ultimately making amends. It was on the third visit that I noticed his intense blue eyes letting me back in.

Within four months (and seventeen years), we FINALLY married!!

My husband is a loyal soul, an innocent energy housed in a muscular and manly frame. Filled with purpose, he has reinvented himself many times over, making him the success he is today. He has a brilliant mind, answering most *Jeopardy* questions correctly and acquiring foreign languages with ease. David is a Grammy-nominated composer. Simply put, his music reaches people's soul, leaving the listener inspired and motivated.

David is as loyal a person as there ever was, as true as his amazing blue eyes. He doesn't easily let people in, but in those precious times when he does, it takes one's breath away. Altruistic to the core, he is a man of service, sponsoring starving children in Africa and rescuing people from car accidents and fires in his other career as a lieutenant in a Connecticut fire department. To know David is to be inspired by him.

I have enjoyed my successes as well. In 2013, I was dubbed the soul-centered psychotherapist and relationship expert by *Elle* magazine. For years, I have helped others to find love, joy, and happiness in their lives. Today, I am an author, teacher, speaker, and meditation facilitator with a thriving psychotherapy and coaching practice. Even with cancer in our story, I pinch myself as I review my life so filled with breakthroughs, accomplishments, and joy.

In the introduction of this book, we describe why meditation is so powerful. Let's make sure you know the keys for a successful meditation practice and turn your cancer ordeal into a healing exploration.

2. Eight Keys for a Successful Meditation Experience

There is not a single person who has embarked on a spiritual practice like meditation, who, at some point, wanted to stop, distract themselves, or quit altogether. The following tips will help you achieve the best results in your new or existing meditation practice.

1. Commit. Read or listen to a meditation every day from this book and throughout your cancer journey. When starting (or restarting) a practice, the natural tendency is to cave in and give up too quickly. Even with the best intentions, about half of you will succumb to your old behaviors of self-sabotage by missing days or even dropping out altogether. **Is that going to be you? We hope not!**

2. Set your intention. Create a goal for a successful practice. This is important. Go ahead and set your intention to meditate every day. Decide that you'll experience great results. For example, your intention could sound like this: *I intend to meditate for at least five minutes every day, bringing more calm and ease into my life.* If you've missed a twenty-four-hour period of your practice, then to help keep you on track, make a special goal of meditating twice as long the following day.

3. Pick a time that works best for you. Studies show that if you meditate at the same time every day, you will have a more profound result. Some of you will prefer to meditate in the mornings when you wake up, over lunch, after dinner or before going to bed at night. Whichever time you prefer, try to stick with it throughout your daily practice.

4. Pick a quiet place in your home, office, nearby beach, or park (wherever you choose) that is your sanctuary. Make sure it's a place where you can't be easily distracted. If you have younger children, make sure it's during their sleep time. Unless you're using the *Loving Meditations* app, turn off your devices and take care of any kind of disrupting noises. Also, some of the meditations in this book are somewhat active, so please choose a place where you can freely move your body.

5. Refrain from giving meaning or judgment to the thoughts, beliefs, fears, emotions, and feelings that **will** pop up during meditation. When they arise, **don't judge yourself.** Gently smile and let them float away. Know that what emerges is ready to leave your system. That's right: all thoughts, beliefs, fears, emotions, and feelings that surface are actually trying to leave your mind and body, so let them. To help them release, be the witness and observer of what arises and watch it gently float away. Even for the most seasoned meditator, thoughts come up. *It's no biggie.* Just notice them with curiosity and let them drift away. Then return your attention back onto the guided meditation.

6. Be patient with yourself. There's no way to do meditation wrong. As with any new practice, patience is your virtue. Be patient and kind to wonderful *you!*

7. If you're using the *Loving Meditations* app, wear headphones. This enhances the sound, which, in turn, creates a more deep and transformative experience. Also, being hands-free gives your body a chance to relax and release even more.

8. Reward or treat yourself. This is a vital commitment you're making for your mind, body, and soul. You deserve to be praised and honored. At least once per week, treat yourself to something wonderful. Decide what that reward is going to be ahead of time so the incentive for continuing your practice stays a priority. Here are some suggestions:

- Take a scented bath at the end of each week.
- Schedule a healing body or reflexology massage.

- Watch your favorite comedian or movie on Netflix or YouTube, especially ones that make you laugh or feel good.

CHAPTER 3
FIVE WORDS THAT CHANGED EVERYTHING

David

My cancer experience began unexpectedly during a haircut in September 2013. Who would have dreamed that a trip to the barber could be life-altering? On a sunny autumn day, I eased into Fast Freddie's barber chair to get the usual. Freddie knew that the secret to a good haircut lies in the symmetry, so he always checked that the left side was even with the right. As Freddie snipped, we talked weather and sports, when suddenly he said, "What's that lump on your neck?" Until that instant, I was oblivious to anything unusual there. I glanced into the mirror and saw a major bump protruding from the left side of my neck. In this unceremonious way, my life-altering journey began.

Cancer was still far from my mind when I went to see my family doctor. The first referral he made was to an ear, nose, and throat specialist—an ENT. I consulted the all-knowing Dr. Google before seeing him, and found a plausible answer to the lump: some kind of benign growth such as a branchial cleft cyst. That was just about within the range of acceptable conditions for me. The ENT doc did his exam, which included my first endoscopy—the insertion of a flexible metal tube through my nose to allow examining far down my tongue and throat. This doctor visit began a period of uncertainty, where one diagnostic procedure after another resulted in no concrete conclusion.

The next step was a claustrophobia-inducing MRI. Back to the ENT. Then a referral to another doc, an otolaryngologist, whose specialty is the medical and surgical treatment of patients with diseases of the ear, nose, throat, head, and neck. Tamara and I went into New York City for the appointment.

This became the most stressful and difficult doctor's visit so far. It began with another endoscopy, but this time I could see the camera's output on a TV monitor. The otolaryngologist, Dr. J., scrutinized my MRIs, and ordered fine needle aspirations (FNA) for the lump in my neck. While waiting between procedures, a sinking feeling that all was not well pushed me into a state of disbelief and numbness. For some unknown reason, the pathologists had to do two separate sets of FNAs. This involved slowly inserting and withdrawing needles deep into the mass in order to capture several samples of tissue to analyze. The pain was exquisite. The subsequent waiting was harrowing. And after hours of anxious anticipation, the five words that changed our lives finally came:

Dr. J.: "You have stage IV cancer."

Me: "Are you frickin' kidding me?"

I felt like I was in a dream state, a surreal movie where my life had gone completely off the rails. Someone had hacked into my life script and maliciously written a terrible scene. I was no longer on the path I intended, as this was certainly never part of my plan!

To be more specific, the mass in my neck was a squamous cell carcinoma. The word *carcinoma* was used by Hippocrates to describe tumors and the finger-like projections that resemble the shape of a crab. Later the Latin term for crab, *cancer*, was introduced into the medical lexicon.

What is the emotional and psychological impact of hearing that *C*-word? Reactions have been embedded in our culture since the 1800s, when the prevailing attitude was *cancer equals death*. Doctors usually wouldn't reveal the diagnosis to their patients in those days because it was considered cruel to do so. Fast forward to the early twentieth century, when surgery and chemotherapy were introduced as effective treatments. Even in 1961, the vast majority of doctors at a US hospital reported they felt telling their patients they had cancer would cause them harm, and therefore preferred not to. By the early 1970s, there was a greater openness in revealing the diagnosis of cancer, and links to environmental causes became well publicized. Cancer remains one of the most feared illnesses, despite modern medicine's advances in treatments, outcomes and understanding its causes.

A lot of cancer information and conclusions bombard us. We are constantly hearing about "the war on" or "battling" cancer, and the message is that we must fight hard, and not give up, or we have failed. If we don't "stand up to" and fight this disease, the implication is that we "lost" the war. The cancer metaphors imply that dying is failure, that we're "brave" or "victims." Even if we "win the battle," we still have to live with disfigurement, side effects, nagging doubts and anxiety about relapse, and new labels like "survivor." We're encouraged to "think pink" and "race for the cure."

What had I done to "get" cancer? A long list of different potential causes scrolled through my mental Rolodex. First and foremost was exposure to smoke and carcinogens during firefighting work. We firefighters are exposed to many cancer-causing substances, like formaldehyde, benzene, diesel engine exhaust, chloroform, and soot, which can be inhaled or absorbed through the skin.

In a study done by the National Institute for Occupational Safety and Health, firefighters had a larger rate of cancer diagnoses and cancer-related deaths than the average US population. In the study, researchers found that 68 percent of firefighters develop cancer. The rate for the general population is about 22 percent. Cancers among firefighters are mostly oral, digestive, urinary, and respiratory.

For the general population, an estimated 63,030 people were expected to develop head and neck cancer in 2016.

My secondary mental list of causes was a compilation of TV news reports and magazine articles I'd seen over the years: cell phones, processed meat, air pollution, radon, microwave ovens, grilled meat, Teflon, hormones in dairy, artificial sweeteners, the sun, silver amalgam fillings, fluoride toothpaste, and even vitamins.

My reaction to the stage IV diagnosis was anger and shock. I'd always taken exceptionally good care of my body. I'm the guy who has the stellar reputation for health and fitness! Now some uninvited, evil poison had triggered this cancerous growth, and allowed it to travel into my lymph system. I hadn't even known or felt it happening. In my stunned disbelief of this situation, I realized my reputation as the poster child for health, nutrition, and exercise was ruined. Now I'd failed to maintain my good health, and I'd have to explain it to every freaking person in my life.

I felt enraged and cheated. I just wanted cancer to disappear immediately. I demanded to have my life back right now! As much as I hoped this was just a lousy dream, I gradually accepted that I was wide awake.

As these surreal events unfolded, I decided not to resist what was happening. I chose gratitude and allowance as I faced the next steps in my journey. I hadn't consciously chosen this circumstance, but I could choose to do whatever it took to prepare to eradicate cancer. I recognized this was a game-changing life challenge in the extreme. What did I need to do to get my life back? What would it take?

Cancer is invasive and lethal if not stopped; therefore, in the context of a living organism, you could call it "death growth." Thus, I had another choice: do I commit to life growth or death growth? And, what positive result can I get from this situation? I had many tearful moments, especially hearing Tamara promise she'd be with me every step of the way. Knowing I wasn't alone in facing this adversity gave me the inspiration to carry on.

In the space of a few days, a lot happened. First, a follow-up appointment with Dr. J. to discuss a plan. In order to begin treatment, the following was necessary: a surgical biopsy of my tongue. This involved general anesthesia so Dr. J. could take a tissue sample from the base of my tongue in the operating room. There was an appointment to meet with the oncologist for exams and discussion of the treatment plan. Back to the oncologist again for blood draws, these to document my baseline red and white blood cell and platelet counts. Meet with the radiation doc for exams and to discuss her treatment plans. Get fitted with a mesh mask to hold my head in precisely the same position every time for radiation treatments. Then get a target tattooed on my upper chest as a reference point to calibrate the alignment of the radiotherapy machine. A simulation of the radiation treatment in a special machine to confirm proper programming of the sequence. A CT and PET scan. Visits to the dentist, since radiation in the mouth area can seriously impact teeth and gums. Get fitted for dental trays for daily fluoride application. After all the schedules and doctors were coordinated, we set a date for radiation and chemo to begin—the weekend just before Thanksgiving.

I was advised I wouldn't be able to do my job as a firefighter while undergoing treatment. This brought me to another opportunity to be in allowance and humility. I decided to address the guys on my shift in person. I asked them all into the firehouse kitchen, and explained to them that I had cancer in my tongue and neck. I told them I'd be receiving treatment and would have to go on short-term disability. I fought back feelings of defeat and failure, of not wanting to miss work, of being viewed as "having cancer," and not wanting to let my FD brothers down.

One of my shift mates, Mikey, took me aside. He'd been through some very difficult times when his wife was severely injured in a terrible accident. He reminded me to take one step at a time, not get overwhelmed, and stay the course with a positive outcome in mind. Coming from someone who'd been through such tough times, it was one of the most heartfelt and supportive things I ever heard during my cancer journey.

This highlights an important point: most people do not know what to say or do when you have cancer. Very few understand the kinds of things that are helpful and uplifting to hear. I found that people who'd been in a similar situation were very supportive and compassionate. A simple thing like a hug can go a long way to show you care if you don't know exactly what to say.

It was important for me to tell people in my personal life about the diagnosis directly. I didn't want them to hear about it secondhand or via rumors.

Tamara and I were exhausted from all the appointments and arrangements. She was also dealing with our son getting Lyme disease at precisely the same time. Rather than calling everyone individually, I sent an email to friends and family to explain what was going on and what we expected to happen.

About this time, I went to see a master at the local yoga center. She wanted to help me with the effects of treatment by attending yoga class and by giving me energy healing sessions. Tamara had been attending this yoga center for years and spoke highly of the benefits. I remained open to the idea, and felt anything that could help me get through this treatment with greater ease was worth trying.

The game of life had radically changed from normal work/recreation activities to being all about cancer. We had booked a family cruise to the Caribbean for December. Now, that was out. We had to find relatives to take our place since the tickets were nonrefundable. At least our kids could go, giving them a chance to have fun and escape winter for a week. Tamara and I would have this time alone during the upcoming treatment. As we dropped off our kids at the cruise terminal in Manhattan, I was disappointed that we would miss the warm weather and the family vacation time. This perspective cemented the reality that cancer had completely taken over our daily lives.

I had made my choice: it was time to get busy living and start treatment.

Tamara

When David returned home from his haircut with Fast Freddie, he showed me the lump, and was convinced he must've pulled a muscle during one of his strenuous weight-lifting workouts at the gym. I said, "Let's make an appointment with the doctor, just to make sure." With some reluctance, he agreed.

Meanwhile, our thirteen-year-old son, Mark, kept ending up in the nurse's office at school, one day with a headache, another day with a painfully stiff neck, and the next day with a low-grade fever. He would feel good, then lousy, and then good again—all in one day. One morning, he showed me the itchy red rash covering his torso, and that was enough to convince me that it was time to visit his doctor. A blood test revealed that Mark had Lyme disease.

I'm not a worrying type, but the thoughts that flooded my brain were causing distress: *Did we catch the disease in time? Is he going to be okay? What if the antibiotic treatment doesn't work? How am I going to keep up with my two businesses and clients when he's home sick from school?* Even though I was very concerned, deep down I knew that we were going to somehow get through it all. However, little did I know that something much bigger was looming over our family, and that five little words would change everything.

Four days after Mark's diagnosis of Lyme disease, I was sitting in the examination room with David while a pathologist used a large needle to extract cells from the protrusion on the left side of his neck. If you took a hardboiled egg and cut it in half lengthwise, that was the size of the lump at that time. As the pathologist walked out the door to take the samples to the in-house lab, he told us both to relax (*yeah right*), and that he'd be back "soon" with some results. He returned in only fifteen minutes, but said he needed another sampling. "Just to make sure." Thirty minutes later, Dr. J. returned and said those five little words that knocked the air out of my lungs. Looking into the eyes of my nervous husband, he said, "You have stage IV cancer."

Stunned, I stared at the doctor with my mouth hanging open. Even though I couldn't speak, my brain was screaming, *Wait a minute! What did you just say? That can't be possible! David is as healthy as an ox! Mark is very sick and you're telling us that my husband is even sicker? This can't be happening!*

David's cancerous mass was growing bigger by the day, so his doctor recommended an immediate plan of action, including daily chemo, radiation, and eventually, if the treatment did not shrink the mass, major surgery.

I didn't know what to do first. Both of my guys were very sick. Our daughter was away at college, and I was the only non-sick person in the house. Needless to say, I was feeling quite terrified and overwhelmed as I imagined the worst outcomes. The unrelenting thoughts of illness, hospitals, doctors, procedures, and treatments were bombarding my brain. Right along with David, I, too, felt anxious and overwhelmed, and was having trouble sleeping through the night.

After several days of this initial reaction, I knew that my fears were keeping me from helping my loved ones. I was not at my best and decided to get a handle on my anxieties. Simply acknowledging this feeling created some relief.

It was time to follow my own prescription for fear by using a process that I had created for my psychotherapy and coaching clients—the method I call *FEAR*. Before I share the process, let's first get the nitty-gritty on fear.

The Nitty-Gritty on Fear

Fear is a feeling experienced when you have made judgments or conclusions about yourself and your situation. Julia Layton, author of the article, "How Fear Works" on the website *Science: How Stuff Works*, writes: "Fear is a chain reaction in the brain." We commonly call this the fight-or-flight response. It begins with a stressful event or stimulus, and leads to the release of chemicals like cortisol, which increase heart and breathing rates.

What was causing my heart to race? The unknown. What I learned in my training as a clinical social worker is that what we don't know or haven't yet experienced, we tend to fear. For example, I've never been a caregiver before, and I was nervous and wondered if I could do it. These were some of the scary thoughts rumbling around in my head:

- I can help one sick person in my family, but not two!
- What if my husband doesn't make it? I can't live without him.
- I'm a bad mother! I should've taken our son to the doctor sooner.
- I won't be able to care for my two guys *and* my two businesses.
- I'm going to lose all of my clients.
- If I take care of David and Mark, I won't have time to take care of myself. I'll get sick, too.
- I'm supposed to be the expert on handling fear, yet I'm terrified. I must be a fraud!

From my years as a therapist and meditation facilitator, I've learned there's nothing wrong with feeling fear. However, fear was taking over, leaving me overwhelmed and exhausted.

Most people experience fear like an out-of-control freight train. The first scary judgment often leads to another scary one, then another... and another... and before you know it, the body is flooded with stress hormones—so much so that even the emergency brake can't stop the train. As you can see with the last statement on my list of scary thoughts above, I not only felt terrified, but I also judged myself for feeling fear in the first place.

Four Steps to Taming Fear

Thank God I remembered my *FEAR* process and began using it when I needed it most. You, too, can feel your calm and grounded self once again by following the four steps below:

F - Face your fear: The tendency is to run away from fear, but facing it creates the courage to work through it. Become aware of the scary judgments you're making about your situation by writing them down or saying them out loud.

E - Embrace your fear: Fully embrace what's terrifying you because, if you resist it, it will persist. To embrace it doesn't mean that you love the awful thing that is happening to you. It actually becomes the stepping-stone toward that thing you've been avoiding until now.

A - Allow your fear to be an interesting point of view: Get curious about what you're telling yourself. Ask yourself if it's even true, which it usually isn't. You can't be in a space of allowance (or curiosity) and judgment at the same time; therefore, releasing your judgments leads to releasing your fear.

R - Radical compassion for you: Have compassion for the one who is experiencing this fear. Tell yourself, "It's okay to feel this way." This is a very loving and compassionate thing to do for yourself, which creates the final release of your fear.

When I follow this technique, I feel grounded and centered. I am able to laugh at some of the crazy conclusions I have drawn. As a caregiver, I'm proud to say I rose to the occasion and was there for David and Mark one thousand percent—and, very importantly, for me, as well.

Chapter 3 Meditation

Releasing Your FEAR

Intention: To reduce or eliminate your fear

Expected Result: To feel calmer and lighter, and regain a sense of peace

We're going to start with three rounds of breath cycles. Each breath cycle consists of inhaling slowly through your nose and exhaling slowly through your mouth.

If you can, place your feet flat on the floor or get into a very comfortable position, one that is conducive to deep breathing. Uncross your arms and legs. Relax your eyes.

First Breath Cycle:

- Breathe deeply into your lungs, expanding your chest. As you exhale, feel all your thoughts and concerns travel down your arms and out your fingertips.

- Inhale and expand your chest ... Exhale. Allow thoughts and stress to travel down your arms and out your fingertips.

- Breathe into your heart center ... Exhale and allow stagnant energy to travel down your arms and out your tingling fingertips.

Second Breath Cycle:

- Breathe deeply into your middle torso (two inches above your belly button) ... As you exhale, feel all your thoughts and concerns travel down your legs and out your toes.

- Inhale and expand your middle torso ... Exhale. Allow thoughts and stress to travel down your legs and out your toes.

- Breathe into your upper belly ... Exhale. Release old stagnant energy through your legs and out your tingling toes.

Third Breath Cycle:

- Last round, breathe deeply into your lower belly (two inches below your belly button). As you exhale, all your remaining thoughts and concerns travel down your legs and out your toes.
- Inhale and expand your lower belly ... Exhale. Allow thoughts and stress to travel down your legs and out your toes.
- Breathe into your lower belly ... Exhale. Release stagnant energy through your legs and out your tingling toes.

Good. You should be feeling much more relaxed and ready to go deeper into the process of *Releasing Your FEAR.*

Take a moment to choose that big fear that you want to release. What scares you the most right now? What are you afraid of? What is causing you the feeling of panic or dread?

If several fears come up, pick the one that bothers you the most. You'll have a chance to release your other fears by running the *Releasing Your FEAR* process again. But, for now, just pick your worst fear.

Releasing Your FEAR:

F is for Face. Face Your Fear - Decide, right now, to face your fear. If you don't face it, it'll chase down until you do, so acknowledge that you've made a smart decision to face your fear.

Move toward your fear and look right into the center of it.

You have an inner child who may be terrified of doing this alone, so visualize your adult you standing behind your child within, as if you have their back. There's no way that you're running from this fear. Facing it brings you both (adult you and child you) to a transformational turning point. Together, you have plenty of courage. You are ready and able to do this!

Move toward your fear and face it. You may see an image or feel a sensation in your body. Maybe this fear shows itself as a color or colors ... or just a sense of knowing. It's all good. Go with what comes up. There's no way to do this wrong. Face your fear, just exactly as it is.

E is for Embrace. Embrace Your Fear - Embrace your fear fully because, if you resist it, it will persist. Embracing fear is not the same as loving the awful thing that is happening to you, it means you're moving toward that thing you've been avoiding ... until now.

Think of small child who is afraid, and you, as the loving and caring adult, embraces that child who is terrified. That's what you're doing here—embracing your frightened inner boy or girl. Use your imagination and wrap your arms around the one who is experiencing this fear.

Be still in this moment as you embrace this fear fully.

Good. This embrace is beginning to release your fear.

A is for Allow. Allow What Is. Allow yourself to be fully present to this fear. Witness it fully, just as it is. You wouldn't judge a small child for being scared, so don't judge yourself. See how deeply you can release any judgments or conclusions you've made around this fear.

Let it go now by breathing in and gathering up all those judgments and conclusions (gather it up, gather it all up).

Breathe out and let the judgments travel down your arms and out your fingertips.

Breathe in and gather all those remaining judgments and conclusions (gather it all up). Breathe out and let them travel down your legs and out your toes.

Have compassion for the one who is experiencing this fear. It's impossible to be in a space of judgment and compassion at the time. Therefore, when you feel compassion you free yourself of judgment.

You're doing fantastic!

R is for Release. Release your fear. Picture this fear being enclosed in a helium balloon. In fact, breathe in and gather all the remaining fear ... whatever is left ... Exhale and imagine all of that fear being sucked up by the balloon. Now, imagine you are holding the string that connects you to that remaining fear. The balloon is now lighter than air, trying to pull up and away ... wanting to float away. All you have to do is let go of the string ... Let it go now ... Open you hand and finally let it go ... Release the string that binds you to the balloon. Let it go ... Release your fear once and for all!

You did it! You courageously faced your fear, wrapped it in love and compassion, released your judgments and conclusions around it, and set it free. Acknowledge yourself for a job well done!

Now that you released it, you can experience fear in a whole new way— FEAR: Feeling Excited And Ready. Go ahead and allow yourself to feel excited and ready for a day of feeling freedom ... of feeling peace. Fear has nothing over you anymore!

Six deep breaths to anchor in this release now.

1. Gently smile as you breathe in deeply, recognizing that you *faced, embraced, and allowed* this ... Breathe all the way out.

2. Inhale deeply, acknowledging that you *faced, embraced,* and *allowed* this release ... Exhale all the way and experience the joy of saying goodbye to what no longer serves you.

3. Smile and breathe in deeply, patting yourself on the back for *facing, embracing,* and *allowing what is.* Breathe all the way out, celebrating your courage to do so.

4. Breathe in deeply, bask in the feeling of elation ... Breathe all the way out, letting this elation expand six inches from your body in all directions, like sunrays.

5. Inhale deeply, feeling excited and ready ... Exhale all the way allowing this feeling to expand twelve inches from your body in all directions.

6. Smile and breathe in deeply, experiencing ease ... Breathe all the way out, expanding this feeling out about twenty-four inches outside your body and beyond.

Excellent inner work! Congratulations for facing your fear and for replacing it with peace. Just drop into your body and sense how much lighter you feel. You should be experiencing more calm, lightness, and a renewed sense of peace. If you don't, no worries at all. Simply repeat the meditation from the beginning and run your fears (one by one) through this process again and know that you will feel progressively better.

CHAPTER 4
TREATMENT: DAZED AND INFUSED

David

For the first time since becoming a professional health care provider, I was required to entrust my health, my life, and my future to other medical professionals. I was fortunate to connect with a trio of doctors who would work in sync—coordinating diagnostics and delivering chemotherapy, radiation, and possibly surgery. I had a strong sense they could produce very good results within the capabilities of modern scientific medicine.

All of the pretreatment exams and tests were expedited. Without actually saying so, it was clear my doctors wanted to fast-track my treatment. Dr. S. (my radiation oncologist) and her nurses informed me that head and neck radiation is difficult, since the beam would affect my tongue, mouth, salivary glands, and throat. There'd be collateral risk to neck skin and dental tissue, as well. Forbidden to shave with a razor blade, I'd need to get an electric razor to accommodate sensitive burnt skin. My dentist needed to be involved to monitor any degradation caused to my teeth and gums by radiation. His staff attended to me with a cleaning, exam, fitting for fluoride trays, and detailed dental care advice.

In addition to these expected radiation side effects, the intravenous chemo I'd receive concurrently strains the kidneys, depletes blood cells, causes neuropathy (a nerve disorder that can cause numbness, tingling, and pain), and compromises the immune system.

The lead-up to my treatment was swift, as my doctors squeezed me into their busy appointment schedules. They wanted to start radiation before Thanksgiving, which was the following week. On Sunday, November 24, 2013, at 7:45 a.m., I was back at the radiation oncology department to receive my first treatment.

My routine, which I'd repeat thirty-five times, was to descend to the basement level where the Radiation Oncology Department is located, check in, and, when my name was called, go to a changing room. There I donned a drab Soviet-gray patient gown. I frequently wondered why they used this gloomy color, when virtually any other choice would've looked more cheerful.

Next, I'd sit in the waiting area, a simple line of chairs in a hallway which lacked visual interest. I preferred going early in the morning, because there were fewer patients and more privacy. When my name was called, I'd follow the tech into a treatment room emblazoned with yellow nuclear icons. I hopped onto the mechanized table and lay supine so the custom molded thermoplastic mesh could be fastened over my face and secured to the table. The tech aligned the external-beam radiation machine using the tattoo on my chest. Then she handed me a foam bite-stick the size of an ice cream bar. Through a hole in the mesh mask I'd insert the foam ice cream bar into my mouth and bite, placing my jaw in a consistent position for the radiation. Now the beam could repeatedly and exactly target the cancerous areas on my tongue and neck with millimeter precision over the next several weeks.

The techs would leave the room and the treatment would begin. I'd try to breathe normally with the mask covering my face and the plastic block in my mouth, and try not to swallow, cough, or sneeze. I couldn't really see out of the mesh; the room was dark and there wasn't much to look at. The tech's voice crackled through the intercom to announce, "We're starting." For fifteen minutes, with my head lashed down and immobilized, I lay there as the machine circled around, calibrated, buzzed, and clicked, dosing me with radiation.

Here I began to experience my first chunk of downtime. Lying there during treatment, I couldn't do anything of a physical nature. I decided to become an active participant in my treatment by using visualization. As the linear accelerator projected its high energy X-rays into my head and neck, I began to picture the cancerous cells as targets in a shooting gallery. I imagined myself as a Rambo-like figure, gripping my bazooka laser gun and blasting the malignant cells into oblivion.

The following morning, I was at the cancer center to begin chemotherapy. Our nurse friend Bettina calls it the Infusion Center, so I adopted the term. Somehow that sounds more appealing. After recording my weight, the nurse took my vital signs and drew my blood. The facility looked dated, well past needing renovation, and the treatment room I was assigned to is small and featureless. The floor, countertops, and furniture were shades of institutional gray and mauve, perhaps once in fashion for medical office decor in 1982. In this small rectangular room were five industrial looking recliners closely arranged. After settling into mine, I was joined by four other patients throughout the morning, some bringing a friend or family member.

Dr. C. stops by as he makes his morning rounds, and is upbeat and cheerful, saying, "You'll do fantastic." He calls the chemo he's prescribed *platinum,* but I know its generic drug name is cisplatin. First discovered by Michele Peyrone in 1845, cisplatin works by binding to and blocking the duplication of DNA. I've been advised of side effects like bone marrow suppression, allergic reactions, hearing problems, kidney problems, numbness, and vomiting. The nurse warns me to avoid unprotected sex, because chemo drugs can be passed on through bodily fluids.

The reality completely sinks in: I'm no longer the healthcare provider, I'm the patient. As emergency services professionals, my colleagues and I respond to help people in their moments of crisis. Our job is to mitigate problems like gas leaks, smoke conditions, or fires. We're there to extricate victims from car crashes, resolve dangerous incidents, rescue people, and treat patients. As an Advanced Emergency Medical Technician, I've provided care on thousands of calls for traumatic injuries, heart problems, respiratory distress, and allergic reactions. I've saved people in cardiac arrest, helped with childbirth, and splinted fractures. Sometimes, the necessary care has simply been offering moral support and holding the patient's hand.

Having started IVs (intravenous lines) on many patients as an AEMT, I can appreciate good technique. I'm hoping my oncology nurse is a superstar. I feel proud of the prominent veins in my forearm and hand, which should make starting an IV easy. This morning I'm looking down the wrong end of the IV needle, as the nurse punctures a vein in my hand and establishes intravenous access. Not bad. She starts hanging several IV bags of chemo pre-meds, a cocktail of prophylactic drugs which include Emend (anti-emetic), Pepcid (antacid), Benadryl (anti-allergic), Decadron (steroids), and Zofran (anti-nausea). The Benadryl makes me feel lousy and drowsy, and the Decadron adds jitters and restlessness to the mix. Behind the scenes, a pharmacist pre-

pares my cisplatin, which arrives in a yellow bag with a biohaz-
ard symbol on it. Dr. C. stops by again, noting that he's checked
my blood work and we're OK to proceed. About an hour into my
first infusion, with the pre-meds on board, the nurse connects the
bag of cisplatin to my IV line and without fanfare, chemo begins.

After the cisplatin has been administered, the next infusion is
Lasix (diuretic) followed by a few liter bags of normal saline solution, to jump start elimination of the meds. This is fantastic,
I've spent the whole morning loading chemicals into my blood-
stream and now I'm going to spend the afternoon peeing them
out. The Lasix makes it difficult to sit for long, because my
bladder fills up so quickly. The nurse has asked me to pee into a
plastic urinal with the ounces calibrated on the side, then write
the amount down so she can track my urine output. I find it
amusing that they've put my initials on the portable urinal so it
won't get confused with someone else's.

On Thanksgiving Day, with initial sessions of chemo and
hydration plus four radiation treatments in the books, I'm glad to
have a short break. Thanksgiving has always been my favorite
holiday, because of family and food. Tamara and the kids serve a
delicious banquet, but the radiation side effects are starting to
surface. It now hurts to swallow, nothing tastes right, and, over-
all, it's becoming very unpleasant to eat. I'm feeling deprived of

enjoying the meal while everyone else at the table is savoring their turkey, stuffing, wine, and pumpkin pie.

An additional week of treatment and radiation has now made my neck mass angry—perhaps even larger. I wonder what's going on inside the lump. Is it growing or dying? Is the treatment working?

Not something I'd consciously choose, but here it was: *cancer*—my game-changing, extreme life challenge. What would this epic adventure be like? Had anything I'd done prepared me? I thought the answer could be yes.

I've been inspired by books and movies depicting true survival stories. I'm amazed by the human capacity to overcome adversity and adapt to severe conditions, stretching the body to its limits. Ernest Shackleton and his men lived through a disaster in Antarctica between 1915 and 1917. While their ship *Endurance* was trapped in pack ice, their expedition camped out on melting ice floes. They were then forced to journey more than 720 nautical miles through Arctic seas in lifeboats. Thanks to Shackleton's leadership and the positive attitudes of his crew for almost two years, not a single person on his expedition perished.

I'd pushed the envelope in my own way. In the past, I'd run several marathons, biathlons, and muddy obstacle courses. I ran stair climbs in high-rise buildings wearing sixty pounds of fire-fighting gear. Twice I'd been to the summit of Mount Washington in mid-January, where temperatures routinely dive below zero, the snowfall averages forty-four inches a year, and the wind velocity has been clocked at over 200 mph. It resembles Antarctica so much that it's a training ground for drivers who will be deployed to operate snow tractors at the South Pole.

I'm fascinated by what's possible at the edge of human endurance. Firefighting is another source of physical and mental challenge. As unheralded extraordinary athletes, firefighters often perform highly stressful and physically demanding actions with no warm-up or advance notice. Calls come in at any hour of the day or night. We're sometimes awakened from a deep sleep when the alarm sounds and it's go time. Firefighters need to have strength, aerobic fitness, and quick reflexes. It's important to be agile and coordinated to perform our job. We do a lot of lifting, climbing, hauling, and crawling through hostile environments, often wearing self-contained breathing apparatus and bulky bunker gear. The personal protective equipment is designed to keep heat out, but it also keeps heat in. Respiratory and heart rates skyrocket while core body temperatures soar above normal.

In 2008, I became a career firefighter after ten years of being a volunteer. I held the unique distinction of being the oldest person ever to graduate the state fire academy recruit program. The Academy included sixteen weeks of military-style workouts,

100-foot aerial ladder climbs, searching in zero visibility through mazes, and dragging hose lines and tools around while crawling through heat and smoke. The instructors gave me credit for performing on par with guys thirty years younger than me.

I ran the Tunnel to Towers race in New York City in full firefighter bunker gear, following the same route through the Brooklyn-Battery Tunnel into Manhattan taken by FDNY firefighter Stephen Siller on 9/11. My buddy Nick and I ran those three miles wearing our insulated bunker pants, coat, and helmet, and, in the process, raised our core temperatures to excessive levels.

My body handled all these challenges like a champ. So I chose to view the regimen of radiation and IV chemotherapy as another supreme physical challenge.

Though the side effects of cancer treatment were so unpleasant that I'd never wish them on anyone, there was power in that choice: deciding to experience this cancer treatment as an Ironman competition: a triathlon of chemo, radiation, and surgery. I was curious: What is my body capable of handling, and how will it bounce back?

I preferred not to buy into the warnings about the side effects I kept hearing from doctors and nurses. I strongly desired not to experience a scenario where I lost my hair, became emaciated, and needed a feeding tube. I was well aware of the incredible capacity of the human body to adapt, repair, and rebuild: the miracle of life growth. On the flip side of that is death growth. Chemoradiation works because cancer cells die from the damage it does to their DNA. Healthy cells can usually repair themselves.

It's now week three of treatment, and I've been upgraded. Bettina, who works at the hospital, must've pulled some strings on my behalf. I'm now on a different floor, where there are nicer recliners, more space, and curtains for a bit of privacy. This floor features a kitchen with a refrigerator stocked with beverages, snacks, and Ensure. Since it's holiday season, there are extra platters of cookies, pastries, sodas, and fruit salads.

My tongue has now been irradiated ten times, and the functioning of my taste buds has become completely scrambled. I'm heartbroken that food not only tastes repulsive, but the sensations are actually painful. Nothing is spared from foul flavor, not even water. It's just a matter of different levels of disgusting. Not being able to enjoy the complimentary food here feels like a cruel tease. I envy the other patients who are eagerly munching snacks and happily ordering their meals from the lunch cart lady. The reality sets in: this is my new life where food = pain. I've lost the reliable gratification from eating. I still hope there's some food I *can* tolerate and perhaps even enjoy. More importantly, not being able to consume enough food has serious health ramifications.

On this new infusion center floor, on my first day, a friendly, smiling nurse named Clarissa greets me. She's a petite Asian who is a consummate professional, and courteously calls me Mr. Dachinger whenever she addresses me. With my healthcare provider background, I totally appreciate her nursing demeanor and expertise, especially her IV skills. She hits the vein easily and painlessly every time. Observing that she pays meticulous attention to detail, I feel more confident and relaxed with Clarissa providing patient care. Her upbeat vibe and positive attitude add a bit of bearability to the chemo experience.

Bettina introduces me to her best friend Diane, who is also receiving chemo here. Diane is funny, with a spunky Brooklyn attitude. She remains upbeat, despite receiving a very harsh chemo regimen. I maneuver my IV pole into Diane's room and we spend hours discussing cancer, treatment, side effects, and potential remedies, boosting each other's spirits while receiving our meds. Diane inspires me with her determination and strength. We forget about our present discomforts by talking about posttreatment dreams of triathlons and road trips to Utah.

Often, Tamara and Bettina come visit for lunch. Their presence is uplifting, like sunshine after a cloudy day. I've begun bringing my laptop and earbuds to the Infusion Center. As soon as my pre-med IV drip starts, I listen to mindful and meditative programs. They help me shift into a better place when the Benadryl and Decadron kick in. Other times, I simply feel too lousy to open my eyes. It's easier to put on earbuds, pull my camo sweatshirt hood down over my eyes, and zone out.

The cancer journey took Tamara and me to places we'd never been before in our relationship. In over twenty years of marriage (and a history that goes back seventeen years before that) we'd never been through anything like this. I believed that I knew Tamara well, but I never truly realized the depth of her commitment. Until cancer entered our lives, I hadn't experienced the full extent of what she's capable of: limitless grace, kindness, and an open, loving heart. As our lives became completely taken over by cancer and getting well, she showed up for me a thousand percent. I was humbled and inspired by her patience and caring. I now had the opportunity to practice receiving the love and care she was gifting me. During this illness, of all the outpouring of support, hers was the most transformational. Today, I'm convinced her love and healing energy played a huge role in my recovery.

It was crucial having Tamara with me every step of the way. The ramifications of cancer diagnosis and an avalanche of medical information overwhelmed me. In my state of numbness and denial, often I couldn't easily hear, understand, or remember medical information from my doctors. I certainly wasn't able to process it, or be present enough to make sensible decisions. I might have retained about 30 percent of the information and treatment plans the doctors and nurses communicated. Thankfully Tamara did, and took notes, which she would later review with me. She attended every appointment, assembling a large binder for all the paperwork and business cards we received.

I was actually in denial that I even *had* stage IV cancer until March 2014, weeks after my surgery. I'd somehow not remembered this label. In fact, *stage IV* means the cancer had metastasized from the initial site on my tongue to my lymph glands. My body had been invaded by an army of abnormal cells that was on the move. The fact that cancer was spreading is what made it so lethal. If left unchecked, it truly is a *death growth*.

Tamara was able to sense what my body was requiring, particularly when I was physically wiped out. With a light touch on my head or by rubbing my back, she was able to infuse a healing energy that helped me through discomfort and distress. Her soothing caress counterbalanced the destructive and debilitating effects of the chemoradiation. Tamara's healing touch became the single most important boost to my body after it had been internally and externally insulted during treatment. In addition, her capacity to love grew exponentially during this time. As my amazing life partner shifted into caring overdrive, I chose to receive her powerful and unconditional love as fully as I was able.

A Note About Friends and Family

Friends and family naturally desire to "help" you when you're seriously ill. Although I was grateful for their generosity and kindness, I tried, but couldn't adequately express to others what my warped eating and tasting experience was like. Some of their offerings unintentionally increased my frustration. Several friends brought over food and home-cooked meals—really nice food—none of which I could eat. Gelato, yogurt, fruit baskets, and soups were delivered. This was tremendously helpful to my family, lessening the burden on Tamara to shop and cook.

There were some interesting gifts and suggestions. A case of aloe vera lotion for my radiation-burned neck arrived and was very helpful. But an old friend recommended cannabis oil and I declined. I was gifted an audio of *Mahamrityumjaya Mantra* from India. According to a Brahmin website, "reciting Mrityunjaya Mantra 125,000 times, will help us to get rid of all ailment & live disease free. It's a boon to sick and aged people. It also helps in prolonging the life."[4] I got to about fifty recitations before hitting permanent *pause*. My dad, who'd been active in the service dog community, arranged for a therapy dog to visit our home. I spent an enjoyable hour with the energetic young golden retriever, who seemed to need calming more than I did!

More helpful suggestions rolled in. I tried to keep an open mind, and read the "blood type diet for when you have cancer" book and took some recommended supplements.

Ultimately, I decided to put my focus and faith in modern medicine to conquer the physical aspects of cancer and also include some healing adjuncts to help ease the damaging effects of the treatments. I was humbled to now have the identity of the sick person who needed doctors, nurses, and loved ones to take care of me.

There were very meaningful and helpful gestures, also. Since I wasn't up for running, my buddy Steve offered to walk with me. We were able to continue our weekly routine of "conversations on the run" by power-walking together. Happy to have Steve's camaraderie, I felt a return to normalcy through this activity.

I'd joined my first fantasy football league earlier that fall and was quickly hooked. Fantasy football became a much needed, excellent diversion for me. My caring friend, Larry, came over

---

[4] "Mrityunjaya Mantra – Heal and Cure from Disease," *Swayamvaraparvathi.org*, accessed August 19, 2017, http://swayamvaraparvathi.org/health/.

weekly to watch NFL games with me. The time spent watching the games together was a true gift.

My firefighter buddy, Tony, paid us a visit. It was like having a slice of the firehouse come to our home, and we had some good laughs. My union brothers donated their sick time, since I had used mine up. Our union officers managed my disability and workers compensation paperwork. My fire department family truly stepped up in our time of need. I was profoundly moved by how our brotherhood pulls together for a firefighter in difficulty.

We were blessed with friends who drove our son to school. Now into the month of January, we were having a particularly harsh winter, with frequent snowfalls. Friends appeared after heavy snow accumulations to help us shovel the driveway. We received an outpouring of loving support from dozens of people. The word spread about my condition. People I hadn't spoken to in over ten years reached out to ask how I was doing.

We set up a private Facebook page to help stay in touch with a large group of family, friends, and coworkers. I posted photos of some Kodak moments of treatment: me passed out in the chair in the infusion center, the IV in my hand, the mesh mask, and a meme of Atlas pushing a boulder up a hill. Even though they were being posted on a social media platform, the daily encouraging messages and posts were immensely helpful and uplifting.

I'd never noticed how uncomfortable I was with receiving support and care from my family, friends, and coworkers—as well as from medical professionals. When it came right down to it, I was resisting being cared for. So, I asked myself this question: "What am I not willing to receive that if I did receive it, would change everything?" My answer astounded me.

For the first time, I saw my cancer experience as an opportunity to receive from others. Family and friends had the natural desire to help my wife, my kids, and me, but at first I wasn't open to this. I learned that receiving from others is a heartwarming and wonderful experience, for the giver and recipient.

The Treatment and My Body

Week Five: it was simply excruciating to eat or drink. The radiation was burning my throat and making swallowing painful. I learned that Manuka honey, produced in New Zealand, was recommended by the National Cancer Institute as a remedy for healing inflammation in the throat and added this into my daily routine.

My irradiated tongue was tender, and I felt worn down from treatment. I decided not to consult Dr. Google about what was happening to my body. If I had, I would have been dismayed to learn that radiotherapy causes the death of most, or even all, taste

95

progenitor cells in the tongue. Daily radiotherapy compounds the damage. Generally, the buds do recover from the insult, but can take several months or years. For some head and neck cancer patients, taste buds can be permanently destroyed.

Though I knew I was eating something that should taste good, the signals in my brain were screaming, "Tastes like shit!" The sensation and disappointment were gut-wrenching. And it was getting worse. There was very little difference in the disgusting tastes of things. My mission became finding something that even remotely tasted appealing. In my search I found that eggs, codfish, and New England Clam chowder were OK. For some reason, these three foods were palatable. Tamara also made me a daily NutriBullet shake, which included vitamins, protein, nut butter, kale, and *love*. I had to drink it though a large-diameter straw to get it past my tongue and directly down into my throat. I could actually feel myself starving as I struggled to consume enough calories. These shakes made a huge difference in my not needing a feeding tube, despite losing a large amount of weight.

I started taking baths in Epsom salts. There was something therapeutic about being immersed in water, and I utilized that time to listen to audio loops from Gary Douglas and Dr. Dain Heer, founders of Access Consciousness. One of the ideas that Access is based on is, "your choice is what will create your future". The audios helped calm me, and were another component of my growing mindful practice during many hours of down-time.

For exercise, Tamara and I took long "gratitude walks" through the snow-filled public golf course. Our routine was to take turns stating something we were grateful for. We'd alternate gratitude statements for fifteen minutes, and it would shift us in-to a space of calm. For example,

Tamara: "I'm grateful that we have health insurance."

Me: "I'm grateful that we have such amazing doctors."

Tamara: "I'm grateful that our kids are healthy."

Me: "I'm grateful that we have loving friends who show up to help."

This simple yet powerful exercise moved the focus off our hardships and onto our many blessings.

As week six of treatment rolled around, my whole oral cavity was radiation-burned. I had blisters on my gums and canker sores on my tongue, making eating significantly more painful. Every day was spent recovering from side effects and mustering the motivation to return again for more treatment. I found the inspiration to carry on, despite the difficulty of basic activities such as eating, sleeping, and elimination.

At other times, I found myself doubting that I'd live through this disease and treatment. One night after coming home from chemo, and feeling the worst I'd ever felt in my life, I doubted my ability to carry on. Feeling frayed and exhausted, I was facing my biggest fear: not living to see my kids grow up, get married, and have families.

In the film *Shawshank Redemption*, Andy Dufresne says: "Get busy living or get busy dying." As I hit rock bottom, I chose to get busy living and do whatever it would take to take my life back from this illness.

Was there an easier path? Curling up and hiding under the covers until this bad dream passed wasn't a viable option. So what other route was possible? I've always loved the quote from one of Robert Frost's poems, "A Servant to Servants," that said, "I can see no way out but through."[5] I became willing to journey through hunger, days of idle time, pain, discomfort, constipation, sleeplessness, weight loss, fear, and uncertainty to get my life back. I focused on being in the space of allowance: a state of not resisting and being open to possibility.

---

[5] Frost, Robert, "A Servant to Servants," *North of Boston*, lines 45–58: "He looks on the bright side of everything, // Including me. He thinks I'll be all right // With doctoring. But it's not medicine— // Lowe is the only doctor's dared to say so— // It's rest I want—there, I have said it out— // From cooking meals for hungry hired men // And washing dishes after them—from doing // Things over and over that just won't stay done. // By good rights I ought not to have so much // Put on me, but there seems no other way. // Len says one steady pull more ought to do it. // He says the best way out is always through. // And I agree to that, or in so far // As that I can see no way out but through—"

Our perspective (point of view) is what creates our inner and outer reality. How I viewed cancer and the challenges of treatment were totally my choice. As an example: I really dislike sitting in traffic. I allow the feelings of judgment, frustration, and inconvenience to create my miserable traffic reality. In heavy traffic, I'm typically very impatient as I choose to resist what is. Thus, my point of view creates my reality. Tamara, on the other hand, does not get upset in traffic. She chooses a different perspective, to be in allowance of traffic by focusing her attention on happy, nontraffic thoughts. She's calm and relaxed. Same circumstances, different points of view, resulting in different personal realities.

In fact, personal realities are the result of millions of decisions, judgments, beliefs, and conclusions. Each of us has a unique point of view, which we've developed over a lifetime. I was astonished recently as I saw this demonstrated graphically. I'd been learning a software program that combines fractal math and computations to render amazing, endless virtual 3-D worlds through which you can navigate. As I tweaked a few parameter sliders, the 3-D world inside the program changed, as well. Several mouse clicks invoked slightly different formulas and calculations, which could transform a cold alien world into a friendly and inviting planet. I realized that this was exactly how we create our own realities: we run "mental software," a compilation of decisions, beliefs, judgments, and conclusions which are the "formulas" that render our personal reality into existence. If we change some parameters, we can change our reality. My mind was blown!

Being unable to work due to treatment, I had a massive amount of downtime. I found distractions like watching *Chopped*, the TV cooking show. I "dined" vicariously through the judges who tasted the chefs' gourmet food. On many days, I felt out of touch with my body. Perhaps it was a defense mechanism to remain ignorant of what it was actually going through. Nonetheless, I made sure my body physically "showed up" for essentials like treatment and yoga.

Like a castaway who can dream of nothing besides returning home, my mission was to get my "normal" life back and do whatever it took to make that happen. All the daily activities we take for granted—performing the job we love, eating normally, sleeping soundly, and just feeling OK physically—I now valued enormously and missed.

In this limbo state, with my life on hold, I committed to stay the course through more weeks of treatment so I could be clear of cancer. My desire to get my life back kept me focused on that goal, but there was only so much I could *do*. A lot of it came down to who I could *be*. With so much idle time on my hands, I could make use of it by practicing patience and allowance. I was gradually connecting with my personal guidance system to help me to find grace and ease.

I also had to be in allowance of the growing list of conditions that I was living with. For example, treatment caused *xerostomia*—dry mouth due to lack of saliva. My formerly overachieving salivary glands were collateral damage, having been insulted by the radiation directed at my tongue. I now had to be sure to have water with me day and night. Certain foods, like peanuts and crackers, would absorb what little moisture was in my mouth and create a choke-wad of gunk I couldn't swallow. I now had a horrible lingering aftertaste. In addition to my sore throat and tongue, I'd developed blisters on my gums. Flossing was painful. The chemo pre-meds created a constant state of constipation. This felt very unhealthy, so once a week I drank magnesium citrate, which induced rapid intense diarrhea. There was a constant flu-like malaise I attributed to chemo. Chemo also caused an acidotic condition, giving me daily heartburn. For some reason, I became very prone to hiccups. I had persistent restlessness from the steroids. Another common side effect of the radiation was thick mucus secretions, which accumulated in my throat and caused me to hack them up. This not only sounds disgusting, but also became a challenge to control. I had to be prepared with tissues and napkins to dispose of the slime.

Here were a few more problems: mouth pain when yawning, facial hair growth wiped out in path of the beam, depressed red and white blood cell counts, and a thin line etched on the inside of my left cheek—a reminder of exactly where the radiation swept during every treatment.

I carried these conditions forward into the final stretch of treatment in January. I stayed optimistic as the radiologist re-measured the mass on my neck. Unfortunately, it hadn't shrunk significantly. As I doggedly completed the scheduled chemora-diation, talk of surgery was becoming more frequent. I wasn't thrilled with that option, and kept hoping that the mass would keep shrinking so surgery could be avoided.

The radiology staff gave me a certificate on my last day of treatment: "Be It Declared to All Present That David Dachinger has completed the prescribed course of radiation therapy with a high order of proficiency in the science and art of being cheerful, outstanding in high courage, tolerant and determined in all or-ders given." Holy crap! I was officially done with chemo and radiation!

Mindful Tip for Chemo

For a great meditation to be watched before or during your chemotherapy treatment, check out "Calm4Chemo" on the *Loving Meditations* app. It will assist you in receiving the most positive experience possible.

Tamara

It was late in the afternoon and Mark was having dinner at a friend's house. David and I came home from a full day of treatment at the Infusion Center. He looked tired and uncomfortable. As he got settled into his chair, I saw him nod off to sleep and decided to take that opportunity to make a mad dash to the market and grab some food essentials for next few days. Within fifteen minutes, David was calling me on my cell and not sounding good at all. Assuring him that I'd be right home, I abandoned the grocery cart in the middle of the produce aisle. I was worried. David never sounded so desperate before. The five minutes driving home seemed like an eternity.

I found David rocking back and forth in his chair with his head in his hands.

"What's wrong, are you okay?"

"I feel awful and don't know what to do," he admitted.

"What are you experiencing?"

I could see him trying to answer my question when he finally said, "I can't explain it, my whole body feels terrible. I guess I feel like I'm being poisoned!"

Feeling unsure how to help him, I asked, "Which part of your body feels the worst?"

"I guess my head. I never felt like this before. It just feels like something is terribly wrong." Alarmed, I asked if he needed to go to the hospital. He quickly answered, "No! Not the hospital. Please, I can't handle going to the ER right now. Just stay with me and I'll be okay."

As soon as I heard his words, "Just stay with me…" something inside of me clicked, which produced a sense of instant calm and confidence. I knew how to help him.

Since David's diagnosis, I had been visualizing myself staying calm, present, and helpful through each phase of his journey. With David well into his radiation and chemo treatments, I watched him get thinner and more uncomfortable by the day. There were many times that I didn't feel any peace at all. Regardless, I stayed very committed to my visualization of being supportive and caring. As if I had a mentor inside my own head, I imagined knowing what to do. *And now*, I thought to myself, *the moment has come that proves my visualization is working! I'm calm and know what to do.*

Throughout the decades, I've worked as a psychotherapist, and meditation and workshop facilitator. I've had to help a number of people quickly calm down from their emotional upset. It was during yoga and meditation retreats that I learned about lowering stress by focusing on the feet. It works like a charm almost every time. I knew David was feeling scared and worried, so the first step to feeling better was for him to focus on his feet.

With that revelation, I sat on the floor next to David's chair and gently took his feet into my hands. I told him to focus on nothing but his feet, especially where I was massaging: The heels, arches, and toes. I instructed him to slowly inhale and exhale while focusing on his feet.

Putting his trust in me, he followed my suggestions without question. *It's already working!* I thought to myself as I noticed his body begin to relax. He lowered his hands from his head onto his lap.

In a moment, I'll describe the progression of simple steps I used to help David reach a sense of total tranquility—a method we later dubbed the *Loving Touch Process* (LTP). However, before I reveal these steps, let me digress by sharing a quick story.

After his treatment ended, David was asked to write a chapter in an anthology titled, **Cancer: From Tears to Triumph.** It turned out to be a wonderful compilation of cancer experiences from patients, caregivers, and helping professionals that became an international bestseller. When he shared with me what he wrote, I was blown away. At that moment, I realized how important the LTP was for him. Here's the excerpt that gave me this revelation:

> I am convinced that my wife's love and healing energy was a huge factor in my recovery. When my body was energetically and physically wiped out, she used her empathic skills and sensed what my body needed. Simply by touching my head or rubbing my back, she infused me with a healing energy that counteracted the effects of the chemo and radiation. Feeling insulted internally and externally

by the treatments, her healing touch became the single most important boost to my body.[6]

Knowing I helped my beloved husband, especially through his worst moments, made me feel very good, indeed. What's amazing, though, is that doing the LTP felt really healing for me, as well. It was a win-win for both of us. And, it's so easy, anyone can do it! Therefore, caregivers, be assured you don't have to be a healing professional to help your loved one feel better emotionally and physically.

The Loving Touch Process

From head to toe, the human body has energy lines called *meridians*. To assist in healing, acupuncturists use tiny needles to open up and release stuck energy from these invisible energy lines. The LTP has a similar effect, yet without the needles.

Bodies typically crave caring touch and attention. The main purpose of the LTP is to allow, give, and receive loving energy between two people. Whether you are the *giver* or *receiver* of the LTP, the goal is to get the energy flowing throughout the entire body.

---

[6] David Dachinger, "Choice and Endurance" *Cancer: From Tears to Triumph,* ed. Viki Winterton, (Charlotte, NC: Expert Insights Publishing, 2015), pages 43-44.

Tips for the *Giver* of the LTP:

- Read over the entire section of the LTP before you begin to give it.

- Decide that you're going to receive a huge benefit by giving the LTP.

- Have the intention that with every inhale, you are breathing in fresh and healing energy.

- Think of yourself as a vessel or container of this amazing energy, first by breathing it in and filling up the cells in your body, then by sending it over to the *receiver*. Think of the LTP as not something you're *doing*, but rather a state of *being*. Your willingness and presence is all it takes for the LTP to work beautifully.

- Important note: Unless you are a trained professional or energy healer, I do not recommend that you touch or hover over a cancer tumor. Since the main goal is to get the energy flowing throughout the entire body, it's best not to focus on just one area.

- There's no way to do this wrong. Your good intentions and willingness are all that are required.

- Don't force yourself to give the LTP if you're not feeling up to it, even if you're being asked to do so. There's a very high likelihood that you'll feel really good by giving it, but it won't benefit you or the *receiver* if there's resistance.
- Always ask the *receiver* for their permission before giving the LTP.

Tips for the *Receiver* of the LTP:

- Read over the entire section of the LTP before you begin to receive it.
- Sit back, relax, and allow yourself to receive.
- At worst, you'll feel the same as when the LTP began. At best, you'll feel very relaxed and much improved. In fact, you'll probably feel so calm you'll fall into a restful sleep.
- Before receiving the LTP, imagine the best results possible. As you imagine it, so it is.
- If it feels too uncomfortable to do anything in Step 1, such as deep breathing or connecting with your *giver*, it's okay—just sit quietly and focus on relaxing your muscles instead.

- Make sure you share your gratitude with the *giver* for being willing to do something so loving for you.

Step 1. Becoming Present and Connected. Instructions for the *giver* and *receiver*:

Breathing:

Breathe in, filling up your chest … exhale and release stress and thoughts down your arms and out your fingertips.

Inhale, filling up your chest again … exhale and release stress and thoughts down your arms and out your fingertips.

Last deep breath in … this time filling up your lower belly … exhale and release your tension and stress down your legs and feet and out your toes … Good, you should be feeling grounded and calm.

Presence:

To help you both become even more present and relaxed, close your eyes, and place your awareness on the cells that make up your remarkable bodies. You have about 65 to 70 trillion cells each. Science reports that 99 percent of each cell is empty space. Focusing on this space is very calming. Be in the space within your cells within your entire body. By placing your attention on this void, you may begin to sense a pleasant light or buzzing feeling emanating from your body in all directions, including down into the earth. As if you have a sun within your chest, allow your sunrays to expand out in all directions by two inches outside your bodies ... six inches outside your bodies ... twelve inches outside your bodies ... two feet outside your bodies ... Keep shining out your sunrays ... it may feel like your energy is filling up the room that you are in ... Even if you don't feel that, it's all good.

Connection:

In this step of the process, you are facilitating mutual trust and compassion. Remember, there's no way to do any of this wrong. If either of you are too emotionally or physically uncomfortable to do this *Connection* step, it's okay. Either allow the other person to do it or move on to Step 2.

Open your eyes and give each other eye contact ... Smile ... Become very curious about the other ... Remain still and quiet and keep as much eye contact as possible ... This may be uncomfortable at first, but stay with it. It will naturally become easier the more you practice it.

Soften your eyes ... Keep smiling ... Become curious and interested in the other. Look into their eyes and say (either aloud or to yourself) these or similar statements:

- I appreciate you so much.
- I have compassion for what you must be going through.
- I am very interested in you, your life experiences, and the choices you've made.
- I'm grateful to have you in my life.
- I admire you.
- You're amazing.
- I love you so much.

Smile even more. Doesn't it feel good to share this loving energy with one another?

Step 2. Giving and Receiving Healing Energy

Giver, ask the *receiver* to sit down or lie face up, however they would feel most comfortable. Using a bed, sofa, or massage table works just fine. Make sure their shoes are off.

To get the energy flowing freely throughout the *receiver's* body, start by using your index and middle fingers on each hand to touch the *grounding points* of their feet. *Grounding points* are midline on the bottom of the feet, between the arch and the toes. Just to give you a visual of what you're doing, imagine there's beam of light trying to travel down through the receiver's legs, but there are blockages to the flow. By touching the grounding points with your fingers, it's as if you are removing the obstruction so the light can flow once again with ease.

For the next several minutes, keep your fingers on the *receiver's grounding points*. Skin-to-skin or fingers on bare feet are best, but socks are fine, too. When I did this for David, I would have him take off his socks and then I covered his feet with a blanket to keep him warm.

Imagine healing energy coming from up above, down through the crown of your head, down through your neck, shoulders, and arms ... out your fingertips and to the feet of the *receiver*. In other words, you are like an electrical cord that pulses with wonderful energy, delivering it to the *receiver*.

- Place your hands softly on the *receiver's* ankles. Start saying (aloud or to yourself) this mantra: "May I be blessed ... May you be blessed ..."

- Inhale deeply and say, "May I be blessed ..." and imagine healing energy cascading down from above and blessing you.

- Exhale slowly and say, "May you be blessed ..." and imagine wonderful blessings being carried through your fingertips to the *receiver's* ankles and surrounding area.

- Repeat the breathing, mantra, and visualization for the next several minutes. In doing this, you may begin to sense a buzz or tingly feeling from your fingertips. This is great. Even if you don't sense this, all is well. This not only *feels* good for both of you, but also *is* good for both of you.

- Now, move your hands up and softly place them on the *receiver's* knees. For the next few minutes, repeat the breathing, mantra, and visualization.

- Inhale and say, "May I be blessed ..." and imagine healing energy cascading down from above and blessing you.

- Exhale and say, "May you be blessed ..." and imagine wonderful blessings being carried through your fingertips to the *receiver's* knees and surrounding area. Notice how good it feels to do this, how calming and relaxing it is.

- Next, softly place your hands on the *receiver's* abdomen. For the next few minutes, repeat the breathing, mantra, and visualization.

- Inhale and say, "May I be blessed ..." and imagine healing energy cascading down from above and blessing you.

- Exhale and say, "May you be blessed ..." and imagine wonderful blessings being carried through your fingertips to the *receiver's* tummy and surrounding area.

- Now, softly place your hands on the *receiver's* heart. For the next few minutes, repeat the breathing, mantra, and visualization.

- Inhale and say, "May I be blessed ..." and imagine healing energy cascading down from above and blessing you.

- Exhale and say, "May you be blessed ..." and imagine wonderful blessings being carried through your fingertips to the *receiver's* chest and surrounding area.

- Next, softly place your hands under the *receiver's* neck. For the next few minutes, repeat the breathing, mantra, and visualization.

- Inhale and say, "May I be blessed ..." and imagine healing energy cascading down from above and blessing you.

- Exhale and say, "May you be blessed ..." and imagine wonderful blessings being carried through your fingertips to the *receiver's* neck and surrounding area.

- Smile as you sense even more blessings coming your way.

- Softly place your hands on the crown of the *receiver's* head. For the next few minutes, repeat the breathing, mantra, and visualization:

- Inhale and say, "May I be blessed ..." and imagine healing energy cascading down from above and blessing you.

- Exhale and say, "May you be blessed ..." and imagine wonderful blessings being carried through your fingertips to the *receiver's* head and surrounding area.

You've done such an amazing job! Feel good for what you've done for you and your loved one. Be grateful for your willingness to do this. Whether you felt energy flowing or not, the fact is, you were very helpful, so please acknowledge yourself for a job well done!

CHAPTER 5
TURNING CHALLENGES INTO GIFTS

David

I learned four brand new things in high school that had profound, lasting effects on me. They resulted from an opportunity to join the track team. These lessons would come into play many times during my life, especially during my cancer journey. They are:

1. Don't buy into your perceived limitations,
2. Go through life's open doors,
3. Embrace opportunities to move outside your comfort zone,
4. Make a 100 percent commitment to anything that is important to you.

Growing up, I was never a team-sports guy. I was more comfortable playing music and reading books. When my good friend Steven, a track and cross-country athlete, suggested I join the high school track team, my immediate reaction was, "Hell no, I could never do that!" The concept of enjoying running, let alone competing on a school team, was way out of my comfort zone. Then an inner voice whispered, *Go through the open door!* I honored that voice, suspending fear and uncertainty, and showed

119

up for tryouts. Our high school track team was blessed with a dynamic leader, Coach Paul L. He ultimately became the winningest boys and girls track coach in New York state history, with over seven hundred wins. During our seasons under his leadership, he showed our team how to make a commitment to excellence and move beyond pain and discomfort.

At track practice, I learned how to push outside my comfort zone and exceed my expectations of what was possible. Previously, I'd never run more than the half a mile required in gym. Eventually Coach L. had me running many strenuous intervals on the track every afternoon at practice, or running down to Jones Beach and back—about ten miles each way! Practice was difficult, painful, and exhausting. During workouts and track meets, Coach would shout encouragement, "Come on, Dachinger! Kick it!" I discovered new personal determination and ability. I then comprehended the concrete results of all my hard work: I became a good runner, began to love competing, and enjoyed being part of a team.

These values later helped me to commit to training and running in a pair of New York City marathons. First, I had to overcome another one of my limiting beliefs.

Living in Manhattan in the 1980s, I became a spectator fan of the New York City Marathon. I would line up on Central Park South to see Alberto Salazar, Grete Waitz, and thousands of runners make the final push towards the finish line in the park. I would think, *I could never run a marathon!* A pattern was emerging. A few years later, I went through another open door, made a 100 percent commitment to training, and finished my second New York City Marathon in the top 7 percent of all runners.

Running a marathon proficiently is dependent on training the body and the mind. The body needs to be conditioned to endure 26.2 miles of constant effort while maintaining a certain pace, and the mind has to be capable of overriding the physical and mental signals telling you to "Stop!" This usually occurs at mile twenty, when you hit the wall. There's a collective collapse of the body and brain systems. The will to continue is eroded. Either the brain works and the legs quit, or vice versa. This is the moment when deep determination must override the signals screaming, "Quit!" It's essentially a mind over matter situation. As the joke goes, if you don't mind, it doesn't matter. In fact, quieting the mind was essential for me getting past the wall and finishing the marathon.

This is when we must tune out the internal and external messages that are taunting us to give up. We must become hyperfocused on a singular goal and do whatever it takes to reach it. We can remind ourselves that this too shall pass and put our total attention on the prize at the end of our arduous task, whether it is reaching the marathon finish line or completing our cancer treatment. We can also concentrate on taking just one step at a time, accomplishing one small manageable interval. This can shift us from feeling overwhelmed into possibility. We can cultivate an inner potency that grows stronger the more difficult our external circumstances become.

I discovered a mindful technique while running long distance that was incredibly effective. I'd allow my total attention to be on a runner in front of me and zone out on their stride and forward movement. This took my focus off of my own tiredness or discomfort, and enabled me to relax into a more efficient, floating stride. Instead of efforting each step of the way, my body had the opportunity to go on autopilot. All systems carried on with greater ease—simply breathing and striding. My mind entered chill mode as I put my complete awareness on the runner ahead and reeled them in.

What do we believe is possible (collectively and individually), and how does that limit our reality? There are many great examples, including that of the four-minute mile. Until May 6, 1954, the record for running the fastest mile had stood for nine years at 4:01.4, and it was believed the human body wasn't capable of running any faster. Roger Bannister didn't allow this perceived barrier to limit his beliefs or his reality, and broke through with a time of 3:59.4. Within the next three years, sixteen other runners also ran sub-four-minute miles once they, too, believed a sub-four-minute mile was possible.

Looking back, refusing to buy limiting beliefs and going through life's open doors helped create paradigm shifts for me. Being a musician, the concept of me joining the local volunteer fire department was something I'd normally never have considered. Then I was invited by a neighbor to watch a training drill, but I was ambivalent, since I had no prior interest in firefighting. I decided to go through that next door to observe something I'd never previously contemplated doing.

Although I was feeling a bit outside my comfort zone at first, I kept coming back to drills and joined the fire company, never dreaming it would become one of my life's biggest passions, and ultimately one of my careers. If I'd never ventured through that portal and outside my familiar world, I would have missed some of the most amazing experiences I've ever had.

Later on, I learned I could apply for a job as a career firefighter. The door was again swinging open, but I'd have to leave the sanctuary of my beloved volunteer fire company, where I had eventually become captain and developed many close friendships.

I proceeded to put my total focus into getting hired, which involved rounds of testing, attending the recruit academy, and paying my dues as a "probie" (probationary) career firefighter.

Fast-forward nine years and postcancer. In 2016, an opportunity came to test for promotion to lieutenant in my department. I could think of a hundred reasons why I wasn't a good choice. On this occasion, I needed some outside validation by officers on our job to convince me to apply for the promotion. Through this open door, I again ventured out of my happy place, as the promotion would mean transfer off a wonderful shift that was like a second family. As had become my style, I put 100 percent effort into mastering the written and oral tests, let go of attachment to the outcome, and ultimately ranked #1 out of all the candidates, clinching the promotion. Now, being a lieutenant is a terrific job, more rewarding and fulfilling than I ever could have imagined it would be.

Each and every time these opportunities arose, my first thought was, *I could never be, do or have that! I'm not good enough, worthy enough or just not ready.* This would be followed by a subtle knowing: *All is well. Just go through the open door!* Without fail, what lies on the other side of that entryway proves to be one of life's most incredible and transformational experiences.

What does it mean to be 100 percent committed? It's the willingness to do anything and everything required to reach your goal. If your goal is to heal from a major illness like cancer, what choices are you making to support that goal? As a cancer patient, caregiver, or survivor, what actions are you taking to heal physically and spiritually?

Are you 100 percent committed to your treatment plan and supporting your body through treatment? The side effects of traditional cancer treatment can range from uncomfortable to excruciating. They can take a toll on your vitality and energy. Seeking out emotional and physical support systems is crucial.

Are you 100 percent committed to living? I certainly had my doubts about three weeks into treatment. I thought, *Why is this happening to me? Am I going to die? What will it look like if I'm not here for my wife and kids? Is that the reality I truly desire?* I considered all this as I spent hours in the Infusion Center with fellow patients, who were probably facing similar crises.

Of course, there's always a choice in how we approach our challenges. I chose to ask questions like, *What is the gift in this?* One gift, I realized, was the opportunity to press the *reset* switch after having such an extreme experience, perhaps the most extraordinary of my life. Resetting is a unique opportunity to take personal inventory and make positive changes. Some lifelong habits I'd developed, like not always speaking my truth, could be discarded. Appreciation for life and living could be increased. New insights could be parlayed into new behaviors and actions.

I asked more questions and made more choices: *How am I viewing my body through this experience? Am I judging myself because my body has cancer? What does having cancer mean to me?* The more I asked questions, the more the answers came.

I initially saw myself as a victim of an illness that kept me from living the life I was used to and felt entitled to. I sometimes viewed myself as a victim of cancer. After all, cancer now prevented me from working, eating, sleeping, tasting, and enjoying life. What constructive purpose could this serve? Certainly, I could wallow in the muck of feeling crappy and missing out on life. Instead, I opted to look for the gifts in the challenge, and make it a journey of exploration, transformation, and self-discovery. Eventually, I was able to take a holistic view of my extreme experience, finding lessons to take away from all of it.

More questions I considered: *Who am I being as I face the greatest challenges of my life? Am I feeling worthy or unworthy of being here on earth? And if I am choosing unworthiness, what am I dying to get out of, by having cancer?*

I believe that during moments of overcoming difficulty and handling adversity, *who* we are being is everything. It's one of the very few things we actually have control over. In those moments, we can grow exponentially. We can learn how to bounce back as stronger, more compassionate people. By bending but not breaking, we can develop grace and humility, which changes our perspective about living. If we approach life's biggest challenges by opening our hearts and being brutally honest, those challenges can turn into gifts.

The De La Salle football team held the greatest streak in high school sports history, with 151 consecutive wins starting Dec. 7, 1991, until the streak was snapped Sept. 4, 2004. In the film *When the Game Stands Tall*, De La Salle coach Bob Ladouceur stated he felt that the team's greatness wouldn't be proven until the mega-streak ended. He encouraged his players to reveal their resilience and be remembered for making a comeback from the adversity of losing "the streak".

My personal winning streak was decades of excellent health. The cancer diagnosis felt like an abrupt end to that run. How I'd choose to deal with it would help define the new me and the new normal.

The cancer journey can be an opportunity to discovery our strength. Now that a lifetime of normalcy has been interrupted, we must face and embrace a new reality. The new normal includes feeling different than we used to, processing tons of medical information, noticing changes in how people treat us, undergoing endless tests/scans/exams/procedures, pain and discomfort, loss of body functions, loss of hair, loss of appetite, insertion of medical devices, surgical removal of body parts, and perhaps, surgical reconstruction. The new normal requires us to embody a level of grit, determination, and allowance never before needed.

I had a deep knowing that this cancer experience was part of a bigger picture, and understood that gifts can be found in any challenge. I was blessed to have lived through stage IV cancer up to this point. If the mass in my neck continued to shrink enough over the next six weeks, I'd be able to get back to my life!

During treatment, the weeks passed, but the mass hadn't shrunk enough. As it turned out, cancer wasn't through with me yet. My doctors advised that it would be in my best interests to have the surgery.

How I Overcame *Scanxiety* with Total Focus Breath Technique

My oncologist ordered an MRI. While scheduling my scan, the nurse asked me "Any allergies?" I had once had a reaction to multiple bee stings, so she instructed me to take a steroid medication in case of an allergic response to the IV contrast agent. Per directions, I took the steroids the night before. On the morning of the scan, the steroids made me hyper and jittery. On arrival at the scan facility, I mentioned to the tech that I'd taken the steroids. She responded that it had been totally unnecessary, since I'd never had an *anaphylactic* reaction to bees. The MRI machine can be a claustrophobic, noisy, cold tunnel that you are stuck in for about forty-five minutes. There's no way you can just climb out. Even under normal circumstances, some people need to be sedated to get through the scan without panic. Now, thanks to the strong meds I'd taken, once inside the MRI machine, my heart began racing and I was ready to tell the tech I couldn't stay in there.

Not one to easily give up, I remembered to put my entire attention on my breath. Since the mind can't focus on more than one thing at a time, this would take my attention off the panicky thoughts about being trapped in the machine. I simply put 100 percent attention on my inhale, and 100 percent attention on my exhale. Again. Over and over. That's it; I focused on my breathing and absolutely nothing else. After a minute, I was no longer in panic mode, and was able to stay calm for the duration of the scan. This simple technique can be done anytime by anyone who needs to get centered and calm quickly. It's also helpful for falling asleep.

Mindful Tip: Staying Present Through Your Challenges

This tip will help shift your attention from your inner world (pain, discomfort, etc.) to outside of you. Find something in your environment that attracts your attention, such as an interesting object, a cloud, a flower or a plant. Silently observe its details. For example, what is its color, shape, size, weight or texture? Don't make a decision or judgment about the object. Instead, be curious and simply describe it to yourself in detail. Once you are done with that object, move on to something else in your environment that interests you and describe it to yourself. Continue doing this technique until you feel more present and calm.

Tamara

There was a period of weeks during David's treatment for cancer and Mark's treatment for Lyme disease that I was running at full speed. It felt I was burning the candle at both ends. There were many days I would fall into bed at night completely exhausted. Regardless, I stayed committed not only to my sick guys but also to my self-care practices.

During this busy time, a typical day began with me waking early and writing in my gratitude journal. For example, I would write statements like, "I'm grateful: we're halfway through the treatment phase; the nurse was so helpful to us yesterday; and, for David's unwillingness to give up."

Next, I would dress for the winter cold and head outside with a snow shovel in hand. I wanted to make sure the driveway was free of ice and snow so David could safely make his way to the car for his morning drive to receive radiation. Since I had to take Mark to school, David had to go to these treatments on his own. I didn't always get a chance to do yoga, so shoveling snow and de-icing the cars were a great way to move my body and wake up. Sometimes, I would walk out to find our wonderful friends already shoveling our driveway. Seeing them always warmed my heart.

Then, time for washing up. Showering has always been my go-to for de-stressing and me time. As a mindfulness exercise, I'd purposely focus on the water and how it feels as it cascaded over my head and body. Numerous studies show the link between water and its ability to create calm from stress and being overwhelmed, which it certainly did for me. If I didn't have a ton of things to do, I could spend hours lingering in the shower or bath. Ah, well, time for the next step in my morning routine.

Next was food preparation. First, I would make Mark's favorite PB&J sandwich for his lunch, and hot oatmeal for our breakfast. Then, I would make and pack a healthy smoothie for David so he'd have nourishment at the Infusion Center. The radiation made the simple act of swallowing a nearly insurmountable task. With each smoothie I made, it took David several hours to drink only half. Determined not to get a feeding tube, he forced himself to drink what he could, one excruciating swallow at a time.

Getting Mark up and ready for school was the next step in my routine. This often included homework that he hadn't finished the night before. During breakfast, I would make sure he took his antibiotic and probiotic for the Lyme disease.

Breakfast has always been my favorite meal, because the kids and I began a tradition of playing games. It started with addition and subtraction flash cards (a fun activity that helped with their mathematical skills), which then led to card and board games. Year after year, playing games helped to keep things light and fun.

By 9 a.m., I would drop Mark off at his middle school and make my way over to meet David at the Infusion Center. I want-

ed to be there for him while he got his cocktail of IV meds—
including chemo.

On Mondays, Wednesdays, and Fridays, David insisted that I
attend my yoga classes so I wouldn't get burned out. I'm so
grateful for his support in this, because during these workouts I
allowed not only a physical release, but also an emotional one.

Since I had been attending classes at my yoga center for so
many years, I had become good friends with the instructors (referred to as *masters*) and many of the other attendees. My classes
taught an unusual kind of exercise that includes a combination of
tai chi, qigong, full-body tapping, kundalini-style yoga poses,
and breath work.

I had let them in on what was going on with my guys and
they freely gave their support by letting me cry during the
workouts. With a tissue in hand, it wasn't unusual for Master Jo
to tenderly wipe a tear from my cheek while I was holding a difficult pose. I remain eternally grateful for all of the support I received at my yoga center during this treatment phase.

Feeling revitalized, I'd make my way back to the Infusion
Center to be with David. I would use car travel time as an opportunity to call my supportive friends and family. These conversations were very important to me, as I received the care and nurturing that I needed.

At around 11 a.m., David was either zoning out or listening to a mindfulness audio on his laptop. I took that opportunity to walk, weather permitting, to the local restaurant to get him one of the few things he could eat, clam chowder, and lunch for myself. Our friend, Bettina, would often join us at David's chair for lunch. She worked in the building next door and used her lunch hour to visit with us and her best friend, Diane, who was also receiving chemo. Since Bettina and Diane are nurses, they were also friends with Clarissa, David's favorite nurse on the floor. As a result, we all became very good friends and have since socialized regularly.

Bettina is reassuring, authentic, and upbeat. She was always patient and supportive with our many questions about anything medical. Ever helpful and available, Bettina became our rock. At the same time, she kept us in stitches. She has a hysterically funny way of telling on herself. "Yeah, I can't believe I just said that," she'd admit while sharing one of her stories.

Diane was going through a terrible round of chemo that left her feeling worse than ever before. Regardless, she was always optimistic, hopeful, and one of the funniest women we know. The mixture of her Brooklyn accent and storytelling skills left us practically on the floor in laughter.

Clarissa is quiet, self-effacing, and always smiling. Just being in her presence makes people feel good. She is truly one of the kindest people on this planet—so tireless, giving, and unassuming. She is the best of the best in her skills as a nurse and as a friend.

Thank God for this amazing group of friends who made the treatment phase more bearable!

Since I work with clients via phone, FaceTime or Skype, it wasn't unusual for me to schedule sessions during David's usual nap time. I had many tele-sessions in my Honda Accord in the hospital's parking garage. Once in a while, I'd find a quiet corner near a window at the Infusion Center. I worried that my business would go south during this time of care giving, but it never did. My clients were all so understanding, and thankfully wanted to continue on the path of their own personal growth.

By 3:00 p.m., I'd drive back to the middle school to pick up Mark and run an errand or two, such as a visit to his Lyme doctor, the supermarket, or the pharmacy to pick up their prescriptions. Because they were always eager to help, I would sometimes ask friends to pick up Mark, so I could either spend more time with David at the Infusion Center or squeeze in more sessions with clients. What a godsend our friends are!

With David's new aversions to food and Mark's unending upset stomach—a side effect of the antibiotics he had to take—I spent a lot of mental energy and time trying to determine what meals to prepare for my two guys. I'd stand in the produce aisle trying to figure out what ingredients to buy for David's smoothies and soups, and Mark's dinners. In spite of my many efforts,

---

Tip for Caregivers

Be mindful of what you eat. Try to eat three meals per day with plenty of pesticide-free vegetables, antibiotic-free proteins, and whole grains. The more you can stay away from processed foods, the better. Don't forget to drink plenty of water, too. Your body will thank you for it during this stressful time.

---

we all ate very little during those months. Along with David and Mark, I, too, lost weight, yet made sure that what I put in my mouth was high quality food.

Evenings were spent attending to Mark and David's needs, which often fulfilled my own. Cuddling with David on the couch while watching the TV food show, *Chopped,* and bantering with Mark during an occasional dinnertime board game, was always so nice. I would use these times as an opportunity to bathe them in my love.

Nighttime routines also included helping Mark with his homework while snacking. He liked my homemade smoothies, especially if they had chocolate in them. I would secretly slip in some leafy greens without him even knowing. Haha, another sneaky Mom who got one over on a picky eater!

One evening, Mark walked into the kitchen just as I was putting some kale into his drink. He was not happy at first, then realized that he'd been downing these delicious concoctions all along. With a sigh and a shrug of his shoulders, he accepted this knowledge and drank his smoothie anyway. *Whew!* I thought to myself. *Saved by chocolate!*

Every night, as I drifted off into my own much-needed sleep, I would imagine both of my guys being blasted with a snowfall of twinkling and healing love. It felt good for me to do this, and became the thing I looked forward to at the end of each day. It was my own version of my nighttime meditation. Making time to go within had been crucial for maintaining my own health and sanity during this challenging time.

Angels

I remember this one night where I was particularly wiped out. Throughout the day, David was feeling quite miserable and I was very worried about him. Sometimes I knew what to do, but other times his agony made me feel quite helpless. Almost in tears, I got into bed and asked, "Angels, if you're out there, please give me a sign that we're all going to be okay."

What happened the next morning astounded me.

It was a bitterly cold day and I was getting ready to de-ice my car's windows so I could take Mark to school. And there, on my windshield, was the most amazing work of art I'd ever seen. Etched into the frosty window were hundreds of perfectly formed feathers. My jaw dropped in amazement as I soaked in the beauty and magnificence of this detailed design. The morning sun was beaming so brightly and directly onto this icy sketch, it sparkled with a pure white radiance.

Wanting to make sure I wasn't just seeing things, I quickly ran into the house and woke Mark saying, "Oh my God, you have to see this!" He immediately jumped out of bed, dressed, and met me in the driveway. He, too, couldn't believe what he was seeing.

We checked the windshield of David's car, but his was just frosted over with no design. Mark grabbed my cell phone and began snapping photos. From the inside of the windshield, the sun cast a golden glow, lighting up the feather motif even more.

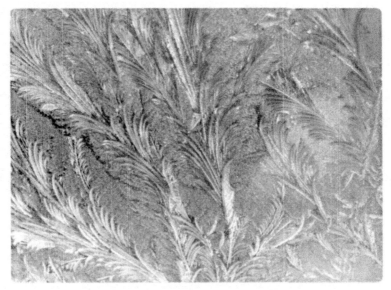

Photo taken of windshield from inside the car

The experience we were having was otherworldly.

Finding his voice, Mark finally asked, "Mom, how could this be? How could such an amazing design end up on our windshield?"

Spellbound, I replied, "I asked the angels to show me a sign that we're going to be okay, and I guess this is the sign."

Just one year prior, Mark told me that he saw a beautiful white angel in our kitchen one evening, so hearing this really excited him. "How cool!" he exclaimed.

We continued to *ooh* and *ahh* over every inch of that windshield for the next five minutes.

One of the most difficult things I've ever had to do in my entire life was to turn on the defroster in that car. We wanted to sit in the Honda and forever gaze at the wonderful gift from the angels. We got choked up and teary-eyed when we saw the feathers slowly melting away.

To this day, Mark and I still wonder in amazement at that magical morning. The blissful memory and message, however, is etched into our minds and hearts forever.

Chapter 5 Meditation

Gratitude

Relax your eyes and gently smile. Prepare for meditation by taking a deep breath in and relaxing all of your muscles as you breathe out. Continue breathing until you feel very calm and comfortable.

Our attention can hold only one thought at a time. Instead of focusing on scary or fearful thoughts that make you feel worse, let's spend the next fifteen minutes focusing on thoughts that make you feel better. During times of upset, you can still find things to be grateful for.

Right here, right now, what are three things you are grateful for?

Are your medical providers helpful? Verbally thank your nurse for their kindness and compassion.

Did someone go out of their way to help you feel more comfortable or at ease? Thank your doctor for their skill or experience.

Be grateful for modern medicine and all the ways it can contribute to your recovery.

Have you thanked your body, for your heart that has been beating faithfully since the moment you were born, for your lungs that automatically bring you lifegiving breath? Every breath you take is a new beginning to each moment in the *now*.

Be grateful to be alive ... to be part of life here on earth.

Be in gratitude for your special talents and abilities, your passions, and your victories over the challenges you have faced.

Establish a daily habit of expressing gratitude. Make a conscious effort to be appreciative for at least three things every day, no matter how small they may be.

Find quotes that express the power of gratitude and share them with others.

Be grateful for the little things that someday may turn out to be the big things ... for all of the beauty you have experienced

... for those delicious moments in the sun ... to live life 100 percent in this moment.

Notice how nature shows up and commits 100 percent to life. What would it take to be more committed to living? Let nature give you inspiration.

This could be your time to commit to life more than ever before. What is the gift in this situation? Is this the opportunity to press the reset button?

Studies have shown that grateful thinking helps you to experience physical and emotional benefits.

Who are the people in your life who have really shown up for you? Thank your family and friends for their caring support.

Be grateful that you live in a time when modern technology performs miracles.

What would it take to be more committed to life? Gratitude is a way of saying, *yes* to life. Be grateful for what life has taught you so far.

Be in gratitude for *you* ... for the taking time to do this meditation today.

Wishing you ease, harmony, and balance.

CHAPTER 6
SURGERY: TOUGHING OUT THE LAST MILE

David

Today is March 14th. It's National Pi Day, because the rounded value of π, or *pi,* is 3.14. But in my world, it has hereafter been designated Surgery Day.

The night before the surgery, Tamara and I stayed in a hospital-owned apartment. I woke at 5:30 a.m. and went for a run through the East Village neighborhood where the hospital was located. It was a chilly damp morning. I jogged my body awake as legions of New Yorkers engaged in their morning routines—buying Starbucks, shuffling toward the subway, and walking their dogs. Returning to our room, I dressed and mentally prepared myself for the inescapable: I was going under the knife today.

Tamara, true to her promise, was a rock every step of the way. She was calm, and her confident behavior helped me feel grounded and optimistic.

I was scheduled to undergo a *radical neck dissection* to remove the uncooperative and malignant lymph nodes. My doctors had done everything they could reasonably do to eliminate the cancerous mass. Because the lymphatic system is a route frequently used by cancer cells to spread and form other tumors, they strongly recommended I have the surgery. The mass had shrunk, but not nearly enough for them to feel confident leaving it in place. I decided to trust their judgment and experience, and agreed.

I had some concerns. Wouldn't removing several glands create a problem for my lymphatic system? How could my body cope with the loss of these vital nodes, which drain and filter fluids and destroy harmful pathogens? It turns out that we have approximately six hundred lymph nodes in the body, with two hundred located in the neck. Knowing this, it seemed reasonable that I could live without several of them.

The surgical biopsy of my tongue the previous fall was a helpful dress rehearsal for today. I was now familiar with all the hospital routines involving paperwork, intake process, and instructions. Dr. J. was almost ready for me. The moment came to change from street clothes into a patient gown, scrub pants, cap, and booties. I was nearing the moment to say a temporary goodbye to Tamara.

Finally, Dr. J. approached and announced that it was time. As before, when he performed the biopsy, he had me walk alongside him to the operating room. There was something very empowering about undertaking the short journey under my own power, rather than being wheeled there helplessly in a hospital bed.

From what I understood, this surgery was a bit tricky. I'd recently been feeling some pins and needles in my left arm, and I theorized that they were caused by a nerve impingement in my neck. There are a lot of nerves in the neck and the remaining mass was enmeshed with my carotid artery. There was also a jugular vein involved.

As I walked with Dr. J. to the operating room, I employed *Ho'oponopono*, which is the ancient Hawaiian practice of *forgiveness*. It seemed an appropriate way to invite positive energy to the upcoming surgery and as a tribute to my body, which was once again going to be the object of rigorous medical procedures.

The simple, repeated phrases of Ho'oponopono are, "I'm sorry, please forgive me, thank you, I love you." They allowed me to take more personal responsibility for my entire cancer experience, and I believed they might allow me to have some influence on the way the surgery would go. I was addressing my body, asking forgiveness, and thanking it. I was also addressing anyone I needed to forgive or who might want to forgive me. It's said we are responsible for everything we think and for everything that comes to our attention.

I felt a bit more relaxed and at peace by repeating, "I'm sorry, please forgive me, thank you, I love you" as I entered into the gleaming, high-tech operating room and climbed up onto the table. I was not totally powerless in that moment, I had control over my own experience, and I felt I could contribute positive energy to the surgery. I had the intention of bringing this state of calm to the whole medical team assembled in the room.

I was vaguely aware that the nurse was putting a patch on my outer thigh. I didn't realize until afterwards that it was being done in case a skin graft was needed for my neck. I watched the anesthesiologist insert an IV in my left antecubital vein (at the bend in my elbow) as I kept repeating Ho'oponopono like a mantra. The medical team prepared to "snow" me into an anesthetized state, intubate me, and perform the delicate surgery on my neck. As the anesthesiologist injected propofol to put me under, I was in a relaxed and hopeful place. Then everything went black.

Many hours later, I awoke in the recovery room feeling groggy but not in pain. I'm sure Dr. J. spoke to me, but I don't recall the conversation. Tamara later reminded me that Dr. J. kept commenting about how much infection he'd removed from the surgical site. He performed many delicate procedures to avoid damaging the numerous nerves in my neck. The mass had invaded the *carotid sheath*, an area where the carotid artery sends oxygenated blood to the brain. Dr. J. was able to skillfully remove the mass from around that vital major artery without damaging it.

One of the major veins which returns blood from the head to the heart, the *internal jugular*, was not as fortunate. Due to the mass being entangled, he removed the vein. I asked about this, and Dr. J. explained that it's not a problem to live without one. In the neck, there are actually four jugular veins to handle return blood flow from the head to the heart.

As I became more alert, I noticed a drain tube sticking out from the front of my neck. My neck now featured a long hockey-stick-shaped bandage on the left side where the incision was. It ran down vertically from my earlobe for two inches, then veered horizontally across the middle, and wrapped toward the front for about five inches.

From my hospital room, I had a stunning view of Manhattan. By nightfall, I could gaze at the Empire State Building, New York Life Insurance Building, and the Citigroup Center tower as they glowed above the iconic skyline. It made being in a drab hospital room much more tolerable. I felt enormous gratitude for the amazing work Dr. J. and his team had done, and felt blessed to have such excellent medical care.

Nurses and doctors came and went on their rounds. I spent a long night with multiple interruptions and sporadic sleep. In the morning, a resident entered my room and slowly retracted the drain tubing from my neck. I was later OK'd to be released. The treatment phase was now behind me.

Hallelujah, my long-awaited chapter of cancer-free life could begin. I felt tremendous relief and a sense of accomplishment. I was officially a true survivor!

Mindful Tip for Caregivers

Close your eyes and visualize your loved one being surrounded by a radiant sparkly white light. Imagine this light is filled with the most amazing unconditional love wrapping itself, like a cocoon, around your beloved from head to toe. Doing this visualization feels good, so do it often.

Tamara

It's surgery day. According to the surgeon, David's cancerous mass had wrapped around major nerves—which could affect his speech if damaged—and his carotid artery. This was going to be a very long and delicate procedure.

As I wait for the medical team to finish operating on David, I look out of the large window of a New York City hospital waiting room. What I see before me is a powerful image that stirs my heart in the most painful yet wondrous way. What I am viewing is the exact location that my beloved may have contracted cancer—at least, that was the opinion of one of his doctors.

How ironic that before me, standing tall and triumphant, some twenty blocks from where I'm looking, is the Freedom Tower. More than twelve years before this day, David went to Ground Zero the morning after 9/11 as a volunteer firefighter, eager to help. His intention was to serve the thousands of New Yorkers affected by that unforgettable event. Unfortunately, there was little to be done and no one to save.

This gorgeous and unusually shaped building represents the death and rebirth of New York—and of America. As it reaches high up in the air, I see how it represents freedom from fear, giving us hope to dream of a future of peace and love. I think to myself, *Isn't that what freedom really is—absence of fear?*

I stood there, reflecting on the experience David and I have shared since that early November day in 2013 when he received the scary words, "You have stage IV cancer."

As I gazed upon the site that used to be the World Trade Center Twin Towers, I knew deep down in my heart that I was responsible for every bit of what I have been experiencing, not only with David but even with 9/11 and beyond. I remember the words of a wise therapist who once said, "If there is a problem, there you are; so release yourself by saying, *I'm sorry ... I'm sorry for all of my erroneous thoughts, beliefs, actions and patterns."*

With tears rolling down my cheeks and with sincerity in my heart, I begin to apologize to me, to David, and to anyone else, for every cancerous thought or action I ever had. I said *I'm sorry* for all things I didn't do and could have; for all the things I did do and shouldn't have; for all the times I didn't speak my truth and didn't allow others to speak theirs; for all the times I judged myself or others; for all the times I ever believed the illusion of being a victim; for all the times that I blamed myself or others for my pain or for their pain. I am sorry for believing the stories of my past that separated me from others and from my own Highest Truth.

The more I repented and asked myself for forgiveness, the more I felt cleansed and free. A softening was occurring. I sensed more than ever my soul being ready to spread its wings and break free from the chains of doubt and fear. I released my past with compassion and excitement. I felt renewed courage and strength to reclaim my life, and burned with love, which was replacing the fear of losing my wonderful husband.

I reflected back on the months of medical procedures, treatments, worry, stress, and exhaustion. Yet, that period also included some of the most touching moments in our relationship.

The surgery took two-and-a-half hours longer than predicted, but the brilliant surgeon did it. He not only removed all the remaining cancer, but also saved the nerves and artery from major damage. We finally heard those wondrous words, "You are cancer free and in full remission!"

Wow! What relief, what joy! How blessed we were to not only have experienced our lives and marriage exactly the way we have, but to then make it through to the other side.

We feel victorious. We *are* victorious!

When you look up and see how far-reaching the Freedom Tower actually is, it's impossible not to feel hope and a glimmer of excitement for the future. It's a testament to the amazing things we can do as creative beings.

I will continue my practice of erasing my negative beliefs and outcomes by saying, "I'm sorry, please forgive me, thank you, I love you." I will do this for myself, for David, for Mark, and for Sarah. I will do this for all of my family and my friends. I will do this for the entire world because one day, I know we will experience a world without a single cancerous thought, word, or deed. I look forward to that day.

Chapter 6 Meditation

Three Rounds of Ho'oponopono

Challenges can be emotionally and even physically painful, not only for you, but also for your loved one who is often right by your side.

Everything in your life—likes, dislikes, passions, health problems, relationships—you create. In fact, you create everything you experience. How then can you deal with the challenges you create? By using Ho'oponopono (pronounced Hoe' oh-poe-no-poe-no) to speak directly to Source energy with the following phrases:

- I'm sorry.
- Please forgive me.
- Thank you.
- I love you.

When feeling disgust, anger, judgment, hatred, or other negative emotions, allow yourself to experience them—it's okay. Then say to yourself and to your connection with Source energy:

- I'm sorry.
- Please forgive me.
- Thank you.
- I love you.

Everything you experience in your outer world, you first experience in your inner world. Therefore, the problems and challenges need to be corrected and healed within you by offering them to Source energy—which is the energy of unconditional love.

As you may experience in the three rounds of Ho'oponopono, it gives you the power to erase negative beliefs and outcomes. As you do it for you, you also do it for others ... and, consequently, the world.

Three Rounds of Ho'oponopono:

You'll get a better understanding of what the phrases mean and how they will release you as we go along. Take three deep breaths to get started. Relax your eyes and lower your shoulders. Say to yourself—to Source energy:

Round 1. Releasing Fear

1. I'm sorry ... I'm sorry for being scared ... I'm sorry for feeling the way that I do. I'm sorry for believing the illusion of fear ... for unconsciously bringing this onto myself ... I'm sorry, I'm so sorry.

2. Please forgive me ... for being so blind when I didn't mean to be. Please forgive me ... I know

that forgiveness is setting me free, so please forgive me.

3. Thank you ... Thank you for helping me. I know
that gratitude is a transmuting energy, so thank
you ... I know that fear is only a projection of my
mind. Thank you ... for bringing me into this
moment so that I can release my fear. Thank you.

4. I love you ... and I love knowing that everything
is love, including me. I love you ... the name of
Source energy ... the name of this experience ... I
love you.

Round 2. Releasing Self-Hatred

1. I'm sorry ... I'm sorry for hating myself ... I'm
sorry for feeling the way that I do. I'm sorry for
making myself wrong ... I'm sorry for beating
myself up ... for unconsciously bringing this on
to myself ... I'm sorry, I'm so sorry.

2. Please forgive me ... for being so blind and not
realizing what I was doing to myself. Please forgive me ... I know that forgiveness is setting me
free, so please forgive me.

3. Thank you ... thank you for this experience ...
Thank you for helping me. I know that gratitude

is a transmuting energy, so thank you ... I know that this hatred is only fear projected onto myself. Thank you ... for bringing me into this moment so that I can release my self-hatred. Thank you.

4. I love you ... and I love knowing that everything is love, including me. I love you ... the name of Source energy ... the name of this experience ... I love you.

Round 3. Releasing Anger

1. I'm sorry ... I'm sorry for holding onto anger ... I'm sorry for beating myself up for feeling angry ... I'm sorry for projecting my anger onto others ... I'm sorry for unconsciously bringing this onto myself ... This has been eating me up inside... I'm sorry ... I'm so sorry.

2. Please forgive me ... for being so blind and not realizing what this is doing to me. Please forgive me ... I know that forgiveness is setting me free, so please forgive me.

3. Thank you ... Thank you for this experience ... Thank you for helping me. I know that gratitude is a transmuting energy, so thank you ... I know that this moment is perfect, just as it is. Thank

you ... I know that holding onto anger only keeps me tied to my past. I am not a victim, so thank you ... for bringing me into this moment so that I can release this anger. Thank you.

4. I love you ... and I love knowing that everything is love, including me. I love you ... the name of Source energy ... the name of this experience ... I love you.

You did a great job. This is your inner wisdom at work. Everything you experience in relationships is never between you and someone else. It's between you and Source energy and it's between them and Source energy—never between you and them.

Recite the phrases in any order. Never say it to another person, just to yourself. Say the Ho'oponopono phrases around the clock:

- I'm sorry.
- Please forgive me.
- Thank you.
- I love you.

To ease your way, have Ho'oponopono constantly playing in the background of your mind. By doing so, your life will be transformed.

CHAPTER 7
SURVIVORSHIP

David: Embracing the New Normal

What is *survivorship*? It's facing a huge life-changing event, and successfully moving beyond it. As survivors, we've broken through to the other side, sustaining our very existence in spite of difficult circumstances. We've lived through and beyond cancer. There's a profound sense of personal power that comes from prevailing over adversity. When something larger than life threatens to overcome us and we survive, being alive takes on new meaning. Recognizing we have the resilience to bounce back, intact yet permanently altered from this circumstance, we approach life with renewed inner resolve. We're more open to new things.

After the end of chemoradiation and while waiting for the mass in my neck to disappear, I was willing to try adjuncts that might help me avoid surgery. I spent time talking with Dr. Dain Heer of Access Consciousness, who asked me a series of deep questions which later helped me develop a new, personal kind of "operating system."[7]

---

[7] For more information about Access Consciousness and the Clearing Statement, please visit https://www.accessconsciousness.com/

Dr. Dain's questions were along the lines of:

- What are you dying to get out of with cancer?
- What is so important for you not to say, that if you actually said it, would allow you and your body to heal?
- Have you decided this is the only way to press the *reset switch*, because there are no other choices available?

These questions sent me further into personal exploration. Are we fearless enough to look inward and ask the difficult questions? And not just once, but repeatedly? Answers and insights emerge more easily with multiple askings of such questions, as we peel away the layers of our consciousness onion.

I wondered how the negative self-talk aspects of living with cancer could be flipped into something positive. For example, I initially thought, "What did I do wrong to bring this disease into my life?" I was now more aware of harboring "cancerous" thoughts, and became committed to releasing them with mindful techniques.

Survivorship also offers us a chance to reinvent ourselves. De La Salle high school football Coach Bob Ladouceur said, "It's not how hard you fall. It's how you get back up." We've faced the cancer challenge. As survivors, we've gotten back up, rising from our difficulty with grace. Now, do we keep the identity of "cancer patient" or move beyond, becoming the creators of our new lives?

I survived cancer and gained a new appreciation for my family. Thrilled to feel better physically, I was overjoyed when I returned to full duty at the fire department and began composing music again. I developed a special admiration for the body's resilient capacity to heal. Having now walked in their shoes, I've become more compassionate towards people struggling with serious health issues.

I acquired a brand-new identity for having "beat" cancer, getting a glimpse of how people viewed my accomplishment when a firefighter was complaining about having trouble sliding his wedding ring off. My buddy Tony overheard and immediately responded, "Dude, are you kidding? You're actually worried about something trivial like your wedding ring, while our brother Dave just beat cancer!" I got a huge kick out of hearing that! I instantly realized I'd done something people viewed as a major achievement.

I wondered, how can I assist my body to continue healing—especially after such a grueling treatment regimen? I began to explore help outside traditional medicine and decided that detoxing might give my body the opportunity to recuperate physically and energetically. After considering several modes, I consulted Dr. F., a naturopathic doctor, who designed a custom revitalization program for me.

His treatment included high-quality nutritional supplements to replenish nutrients my organs and tissues had lost, and to help them regenerate. The huge assortment of supplements included enzymes, zinc, lipotropic complex, adrenal response care, clinical nutrients for men, vitamin C powder, renewal greens, propolis throat spray and herbal mouthwash. I was directed to eat a diet of healing foods, dairy product alternatives, nutritional yeast, Bragg's cider vinegar, flaxseed and probiotics. This anti-inflammatory diet featured organic, low-glycemic, high-fiber and gluten-free foods, adding calories and protein. For the first time I could remember, I actually had to work at gaining weight.

In addition, I received regular acupuncture treatments from Dr. F., aimed at improving lingering side effects and boosting my depressed immune system. At home, to aid detoxification, I applied castor oil packs for my liver, dry-brushed my skin with a loofah, and ended my showers with a cold spray. The theme that guided me throughout was: *Be open to everything that is possible in the world.*

The master at the yoga center continued to do healing sessions with me. One session included *moxibustion*, where a smoldering herb is placed near where thumbs/index fingers and big toes/second toes meet. The purported benefits were increased immunity and improved energy, but the visible results were some minor burns on my feet. The master also performed healing massages and acupressure. I began attending yoga classes, which helped me recharge and improved stamina.

I tried *As Seen on TV - Detoxify While You Sleep!* footpads at night. They'd change dramatically from white to brown by morning. This visual was so satisfying, I lightheartedly figured this color change was proof the pads were actually drawing toxins out of my feet.

I met a woman who does colonics. I was hoping that flushing lingering chemo toxins from my gastrointestinal system would help me feel noticeably better and more energetic. The process was tolerable, but I didn't feel a profound difference. The colonic was followed by an ionic detox footbath. The theory is the water turns a particular color on a chart—from yellow to reddish-brown—depending which toxic material is removed from your body. The resulting hue of the water was a dramatic orange as my feet soaked and the machine bubbled. As with most things too good to be true, I later discovered this device does nothing more than generate rust from its iron electrodes.

In addition to alternative and nontraditional treatments, I stayed true to the foundation lifestyle that helped ease me through treatment in the first place: exercise, good nutrition, sleep, laughter, Tamara's love, gratitude for family, and continuing my mindful practice. Slowly I was able to increase the length and intensity of my workouts, eventually returning to road running and lifting weights at the gym.

The number of people touched by cancer has reached epic proportions, with millions facing the challenges of the disease. According to the American Cancer Society and the National Cancer Institute, there were more than 15.5 million estimated cancer survivors alive in the United States in 2016. That number is expected to grow to over 20 million by 2026. In 2016, an estimated 1.6 million new cancer cases were diagnosed in the United States alone, creating huge numbers of patients beginning their cancer odyssey.

Like an exclusive fellowship, all of us who have lived with cancer are connected. We have a new identity: cancer survivor. There's even a National Cancer Survivor Day celebrated annually on the first Sunday each June.

Our modern vernacular often says we are "battling" cancer. Many continue that battle through social media. Our Twitter descriptions read "warrior husband," "stage 1-2-3-4," "BRCA 2 positive," "Stage IV colon cancer survivor," "Living with metastatic breast cancer," and "Men Have Breasts Too".

There are a huge number of cancer support communities online and in facility meeting rooms. These groups offer support for very specific variations of the disease and for different demographics of cancer survivors, such as stage, type of treatment, and age.

As cancer survivors, we must also cope with the constant uncertainty of relapse. For instance, we may frequently check our bodies for lumps, bumps, aches, and other signs of the cancer coming back. After treatment ended, I kept stretching my tongue to the far side of my mouth to see if it felt normal. Because something internal was removed in the surgery, my left neck now felt taut when I stretched out my tongue. Even now it never feels normal. Welcome to the *new normal*.

The new normal includes anxiety around follow-up doctor visits. As I'm being examined and scanned, I sometimes worry something new will show up, because the doctors always appear to be looking for something amiss. When the exam is over and I'm told everything is all clear, I indulge in a sigh of relief, but the doctor is already booking my next scan and follow-up visit. Immediately, the clock starts ticking down to this future appointment.

In addition, we may know others who've had to return for treatment because the cancer came back. How can we continue to live without fear and anxiety ruling our thoughts? The good news is we have tools to help us live calm with and beyond cancer, so let's remember to use them!

One mindful tip is to think or say, "All is well" ten times. Notice how just saying it feels good, and you begin to relax. Even if you don't fully believe it in the moment, repeating this simple phrase can center us and keep us feeling positive.

As a survivor, I'm totally committed to paying forward the lessons I've learned on my cancer journey. Along with Tamara, my mission is to share acquired insights and information with the cancer community, patients, survivors, and care partners. The mindfulness techniques that helped me live calm with cancer remain vital to my survivorship today. Amazingly, those insights and practices would also play a major role in the next incredible chapter of our lives.

Mindful Tip for Caregivers

Close your eyes and relax. Imagine that you have a large paintbrush in your hand, the kind you'd use to paint a large room. Visualize taking your paintbrush and dipping it into a can of wall paint. On your imaginary wall, paint the number "1." As you dip your paintbrush into the can of paint again, pretend that the "1" just disappears and that your imaginary wall becomes blank. Next, visualize yourself painting the number "2" on your imaginary wall.

Keep repeating this until you reach number "10" or feel more tranquil, whichever comes first.

This is also a great tip for getting yourself to sleep every night.

Tamara: From Cancer Blues to Mini-Blue

It's 3:00 a.m., and I wake up realizing this is the last day with our beloved Mini-Blue. I remember the day when she became part of our family; David, Mark, and I had walked into the Mini Cooper dealership, wide-eyed and excited. Smiling, we all had the same thought, *This day is finally here! We made it!*

You see, this hadn't been any ol' day; this had been the zenith we'd been waiting for, where one dramatic period of our lives ended and a new and exciting one began.

When your son and husband are in the middle of their treatments for their illnesses *and* your Honda lease is up, what does one do? My brother offered to fly into New York and go to the dealership with me to help me select my new car, but David said, "No, that's my job. I'm going to beat this thing, get through my treatments, and be in that dealership with you. We're doing this together, like we always have." That same day, I called my financial agency to extend the lease for another three months.

During the grueling treatment phase, there was at least the sunshiny topic of what car I was going to get next.

My Honda was a sensible family car that I'd been driving for years. It had become the caregiver taxi, as well, driving my guys to their endless doctor's appointments. I dreamed of something fun, different, and inspiring.

Every time I'd seen a Mini Cooper drive by, my mouth watered. I saw each one as unique and colorful. Some had stripes down the hood, while others had detailing down the back. Some were convertible 2-doors, while others were sunroof 4-doors. All of them were like candy to me. I drooled over them and couldn't wait to drive one.

Mark and I would pore over their brochures and website, *oohing* and *ahhing* at the 2-door models while David (always Mr. Safety) quietly pointed to the safer 4-door models. After illness, doctors, treatments, and procedures, planning my next car was a fun and bright activity for the three of us.

There were two big hurdles to jump over before walking through the doors of the Mini Cooper dealership, however. After three months of antibiotics, one goal was to get a thumbs-up from Mark's Lyme specialist. We breathed a huge sigh of relief when the doctor reported that we had caught the disease in time. The medication had worked and Mark was going to be just fine.

With one hurdle down we had one to go: David's surgery. And, as you already know, it was a huge success!

Two weeks later: Mini Cooper, here we come!

So, you can only imagine why that day had been so special, the three of us walking into that car dealership scoping out the Minis that looked like Matchbox cars, each one just as colorfully tempting as the next. This was the tantalizing day we'd been waiting for.

Tough decision, but I ended up choosing a blue Mini Cooper Countryman 4-door (yes, Mr. Safety won on that front). The color blue symbolizes strength and is known to have a calming effect on the psyche. It also reminded me of the sky and the sea, so limitless and filled with possibilities for the future. Mark and I dubbed our newest addition to the family Mini-Blue, our valiant representative of what is possible.

Mini-Green

Fast forward: it's hard to imagine that three years have gone by. Mini-Blue's lease is up.

Both of my guys are doing great and Mini-Blue has been a constant reminder of how important it is to have fun, be strong, and focus on the benefits that life has to offer.

I'm now picking up my new green Mini Cooper Special Edition Countryman. The color green represents renewal, nature, and energy, symbolizing all the best of life. Mark wants to call him Mini-Hulk. I'm more partial to Mini-Grand. I guess the longest straw will win.

I'm not sure what we'll end up naming him but there's no question that the three of us have triumphed over illness and a truly difficult period in our lives. Hmmmm... Maybe we should call him Mini-Victory?

Chapter 7 Meditation

Feel Life: All Is Well

If you are living with a serious illness, like cancer, or are a survivor, or feeling the stress of being a caregiver, this meditation will help you become aware of how life flows and grows, gracefully and easily.

Nature shows that our cells are filled with life-force energy and infinite possibility.

Instead of focusing on our diseased cells, what if, for today, we focus on how most cells in our bodies are filled with life-force energy?

Nature reminds us that life continues and all is well.

ALL IS WELL ...

Feel life ... Notice that life is happening everywhere. Seeing a flower is simply an affirmation that life exists in abundance, all around us and inside of us.

What is the nature of all living things on this beautiful planet? We have the freedom to grow and expand outward.

Life-growth is unstoppable on every level.

Life-growth is constant as the cycle always continues.

Life is growth and expansion.

We share a connection with life on this planet. The quieter we become, the more we can hear. Through this connection we discover peace, compassion, joyfulness, and satisfaction. Through this connection we can express creation and the life-force within us.

Place your awareness on life and living on this beautiful planet.

Plants show us the limitless ability they have to grow, to blossom, to share their beauty.

When the warmth of the sun touches plants and trees, they respond with life-growth, offering us colors, shapes, symmetry, and pleasing aromas.

When the warmth of the sun reaches plants and trees, they respond with effortless life-growth, offering us flowers and fruit.

When we put our attention on nature, we feel a connection with its depth and beauty. That connection helps us to be grounded in the present moment.

All of nature gracefully moves through the cycle of life.

The movements of life rise and fall, always flowing with ease.

Feel life. Notice that life is happening everywhere and ... all is well.

CHAPTER 8
UNSTOPPABLE: *LOVING MEDITATIONS* IS BORN

About a year after my initial diagnosis of stage IV cancer, I had a follow-up visit with my oncologist Dr. C. As always, Tamara accompanied me for emotional support and to lend a second set of ears while pertinent medical information was discussed. After my vitals were taken and blood drawn, we had a brief wait in the bleak exam room. Then Dr. C. entered, crowing in his usual style, "How are you, David! You look great!"

During this exam, Dr. C. announced that my scans were clear and I was now officially cancer-free. He commented, "That was not an easy regimen you just had, but you did phenomenally well!" He asked if there was actually something I did which helped me get through treatment in such good emotional and physical shape. I replied that I'd used a mindful practice, including audio programs. His eyes lit up as he suddenly proclaimed, "That's what I want for all of my patients!"

Dr. C. proceeded to chat about how the cancer treatment center was busier than ever. His time spent with patients was getting increasingly more limited. He wished there was a way his patients could become calm before their exams or treatments.

As Dr. C. talked, Tamara's eyes and mine met. A light bulb lit up. We'd been creating and webcasting a guided meditation series called *Miracle Mondays Meditations* for seven years. A large audience connected with the style and vibe we'd developed. We'd also recently lived through the cancer experience as patient and caregiver. Now my doctor was pointing out a shortcoming within his oncology practice.

Tamara and I had the skills and creative ability, we had walked the walk, and there was a clear need in the cancer community. As we exchanged huge smiles, we had our *a-ha!* moment: *Loving Meditations* was born.

Since we were both in helping professions, we deeply desired to be of service to others, especially those navigating major health challenges. Our hearts were full of empathy for both patients and caregivers. We truly understood their pain points. Now we had an additional perspective: survivorship.

Given the insights we had gained at Dr. C.'s office, we asked ourselves, "What would it take to create mindfulness programs specifically for the cancer community?" Offering videos and audios online was a possibility, and the proliferation of apps on personal devices provided the perfect medium to deliver *Loving Meditations*. We proceeded to brainstorm.

Through the app, patients could view the meditations in their infusion center, during downtime, or while waiting for treatment, exams, or scans. Patients and caregivers usually have significant time while preparing for the next round of appointments and treatments, an interval when they typically need to rest and recharge. *Loving Meditations* would be helpful those days as well.

Immediately, it was clear to Tamara and me that we had a new mission: Bring our mindfulness programs to those challenged with the same cancer-related issues we had experienced. Inspired to take our skills to the next level, we were excited to be a contribution to this group. *Loving Meditations* would offer patients and care partners the tools to become active participants in their healing journey. And for those who had completed treatment, *Loving Meditations* could assist them during the survivorship phase.

We discovered an excellent book, *Mindfulness-Based Cancer Recovery: A Step-by-Step MBSR Approach to Help You Cope with Treatment and Reclaim Your Life*, by Drs. Linda Carlson, Michael Speca, and Zindel Segal. It has an abundance of useful information and exercises for mindfulness-based stress reduction (MBSR) specifically designed for cancer patients and survivors. These cancer-specific MBSR techniques, called *mindfulness-based cancer recovery*, are intended to be used during treatment and recovery.

We also learned that meditation has deep roots in research-based results. In a study published in November 2014 in the journal *Cancer*, researchers led by Dr. Carlson at the University of Calgary found the first evidence that suggests that participating in support groups or yoga/meditation is capable of positively altering the *telomere length* of the cells of cancer survivors. Telomeres are protein caps at the end of our chromosomes and determine how quickly cells age. Shortened telomeres are often linked with diseases like cancer. One group's members were asked to practice yoga and meditation at home daily for forty-five minutes, another group was encouraged to share about their worries and emotions. Members in both the meditation/yoga and sharing group were found to have telomeres that measured longer than the control group.

Nature has a profound healing effect. Studies show exposure to nature contributes to physical well-being, reducing heart rate, blood pressure, muscle tension, and the production of stress hormones. According to public health research scientists Stamatakis and Mitchell, it may even reduce mortality. Research done in hospitals, offices, and schools has found that even a simple plant in a room can have a significant positive impact on stress and anxiety.

CancerNetwork.com, home of the journal *Oncology*, reported that mind-body practices like mindfulness meditation have been shown to "positively affect quality of life and biological outcomes" when used by cancer patients and healthcare professionals.

Let's face it. Cancer and other major illnesses are scary, overwhelming, and stressful. As you've heard from our own journey, it can also be an opportunity for healing and self-discovery. With this in mind, we created *Loving Meditations* to pay forward the huge benefits of mindfulness for any major medical challenge.

The *Loving Meditations* App is available on two platforms, iOS (for iPad and iPhone) and Web App (for any device). For the free app download, go to calmcancerstress.com

For Patients

Imagine you're sitting in the infusion center hooked up to a cocktail of IV medications. You are expecting to be sitting there for a few hours, anticipating discomfort and with time on your hands. Then you remember you have the *Loving Meditations* app on your device. Shifting into calm and ease is as simple as opening the app and answering a few questions with the Adviser feature. For example, when the Adviser asks, *"Do you feel pain or discomfort?"* you may choose to swipe right for yes. The Adviser uses your swipe response to quickly guide you to helpful programs. Next, press play and enjoy the meditation. Whether you close your eyes and zone out or watch the beautiful images on the screen, you'll be transported to a state of relaxation and tranquility. (Note: See Appendix A for a listing of all *Loving Meditations* programs).

For Caregivers

Imagine that you are completely exhausted, overwhelmed, and in need of a recharge. While your loved one is receiving treatment, the *Loving Meditations* app sends you a reminder to watch the next meditation in your current program. You pop in your ear buds and see that the next meditation in the "Vital Recharge" program is *Refresh. Revitalize. Renew.* Within minutes, you should be feeling much more energized, refreshed and inspired to go on with your day.

For Survivors

Imagine you're scheduled for a follow-up scan and are beginning to feel anxious about the procedure and results. Looking at your device screen, you notice an inspiring quote there from *Loving Meditations*. Opening the app, you navigate to one of the *Mindful Minute* videos called *Total Focus Breath,* a super easy technique to use anytime, anywhere to quickly calm and quiet the mind. You follow the breathing technique for the next several minutes. Quickly, a sense of "I've got this" replaces panic.

For the Waiting Room: *Loving Meditations* TV

Our cancer experience made us aware of another stressful problem many encounter: the waiting room. How many times had we gone to meet with doctors, gone for scans or treatment, and had to sit in a waiting area with a raucous TV? Most of the time, the loud, chatty program would be a news show with negative stories and banners flashing, "News Alert!" Other times, there'd be a clamorous talk or game show, with loud voices punctuated by bells, buzzers, laughter, and applause. We noticed people in the waiting room becoming just as frazzled as we were by the TV, the intense messages, and images. There was no way to shut this out, unless the staff turned down the volume or changed the channel.

CNBC reported in 2016 that 63 percent of surveyed patients said the most stressful thing about going to their MD was waiting. As we anxiously anticipate procedures, treatments, scans, exams, or the results thereof, the waiting room TV becomes a source of additional stress. The TV produces an unwelcome assault on our eyes and ears. What if waiting room TV could be used to benefit patients instead of stressing them?

The American Journal of Managed Care estimates that for people seeking medical care, out of a total of eighty-seven minutes at the doctor's office, only twenty of those minutes are actually spent in the presence of a physician. Time spent in waiting rooms is a fact of life for those of us who often visit multiple doctors and receive regular diagnostic testing and other procedures.

Many of us suffer from white-coat hypertension, where the stress of seeing the doctor raises our blood pressure. David was amazed how much higher his "textbook normal" blood pressure elevated during an oncologist visit. We learned that incorporating peaceful scenes of nature with beautiful music has a therapeutic effect, reducing the stress of patients, families, caregivers, office staff, and healthcare providers.

This led to the creation of *Loving Meditations TV*, programs which easily calms the atmosphere in waiting areas. Picture spectacular nature images such as mountains, lakes, clouds, forests, and soaring birds with an expansive music soundtrack. These elements assist viewers to feel more grounded, centered, and tranquil while waiting for healthcare services.

Since our relaxing footage was already drawing in the viewer, we enhanced it with *Mindful Facts*—inspirational messages displayed with the video. These remind us of the amazing abilities of the human body and the benefits of deep breathing and meditation. *Mindful Facts* also displays inspiring quotes by prominent figures about overcoming adversity. To encourage the viewer's active participation, *Loving Meditations TV* provides prompts to activate mindful breathing.

For more information on *Loving Meditations TV*, please go to https://lovingmeditations.com/loving-meditations-wrtv/ .

Outreach to the Cancer Community

As we began outreach and connected with the cancer community, we recognized we could also be a contribution in person. Through live workshops, we present our meditations and mindfulness exercises to community cancer organizations like Gilda's Club and hospital cancer support groups. The immediate feedback from participants helps us develop new meditations and programs. Other outreach includes speaking before groups including seniors and cancer survivors about mindfulness and cancer.

Tamara has produced a series of blogs, available on the LovingMeditations.com website, offering valuable information for patients, survivors and caregivers. We appear regularly on TV, radio shows, and podcasts sharing the benefits of meditation and mindful tips.

Born from the life-altering experience called *cancer, Loving Meditations* is our way to create mindful content together. The opportunity to pay it forward is truly one of the beautiful gifts we received as a result of our dance with cancer. Our wish is to help you on your journey, with ease and grace.

Our mindful techniques worked beautifully for us and also have helped thousands of people in over twenty countries. We encourage you to practice the mindful tips and meditations in this book. Along with the *Loving Meditations* app, they'll assist you to find calm and relief from discomfort. It really is as simple as putting on your earbuds or headphones and pressing *play*.

We've heard folks say, "Yeah, but I have no time to meditate!" Looking at it another way, we don't realize how much time we actually spend watching the news, TV programs, or digital content on social media. Many of us devote significant time to this, sometimes to the point of addiction. In 2016, the Nielsen Company found that adults in the United States spend about ten-and-a-half hours each day consuming media on tablets, smartphones, personal computers, TVs and other devices. How much of that news and other content actually makes us feel good? Chances are, those messages are not helping the cause of inner peace!

Graham C. L. Davey, PhD reported in *Psychology Today* that if viewing a TV program creates negative emotions such as anger, sadness or anxiety, this will influence your life experiences, the memories you recall and the degree of worry you feel.

The news offers a very specific window on the world, and features events we may have little or no control over. Why not put more attention on things you *can* control: your breath, your serenity, and your happiness? Reclaim some of your precious time; quiet your mind and shift into calm.

Another common problem people mention about starting a mindful practice is that they can't stop thinking and their mind is too "active" to meditate. They may have tried meditating in the past and found it difficult to sit and do nothing. Barraged by thoughts, they can't shut them out.

To address this concern, we'd like to reiterate one the Eight Keys For A Successful Meditation Experience from Chapter 1:

> Refrain from giving meaning or judgment to the thoughts, beliefs, fears, emotions, and feelings that will pop up during meditation. When they arise, *don't judge yourself.* Gently smile and let them float away. Know that what emerges is ready to leave your system. That's right, all thoughts, beliefs, fears, emotions, and feelings that surface are actually trying to leave your mind and body, so let them. To help them release, be the witness and observer of what arises and watch it gently float away. Even for the most seasoned meditator, thoughts come up. *It's no biggee.* Just notice them with curiosity and let them drift away.

Then return your attention back onto the guided meditation.

We thank you for joining us as we shared our story and the mindful tools that helped us live calm with and beyond cancer. Cancer and other serious illnesses are extreme events in life, which offer unique opportunities for personal transformation and spiritual evolution. We hope you find the gifts in those challenges.

We wish you peace and ease on your journey!

ABOUT THE AUTHORS

David Dachinger and Tamara Green, LCSW are the co-founders of *Loving Meditations*. David is a featured author and Grammy-nominated composer who has scored inspiring music for America's most celebrated sporting events and television shows. Over 1.5 billion people have heard his music on *CBS* broadcasts of the *Super Bowl*, *The Masters*, and NFL games. David is a survivor of stage IV head, neck, and lymphatic cancer. Tamara is an author, speaker, and trainer, whom *Elle* magazine referred to as "the soul-centered psychotherapist and meditation facilitator." Tamara combines her many years of professional training and her life experience as a caregiver to create powerfully effective guided meditations that have helped thousands to achieve peace, love, and well-being. Together, this married couple has created transformative mindfulness programs that help patients and caregivers to dramatically reduce stress, anxiety, pain, and discomfort throughout their medical ordeal. Check out their website at lovingmeditations.com or contact them at info@lovingmeditations.com.

A Loving Meditations Rave:

I went for my medical treatment yesterday and I am happy to say that I am 100% healed! My doctor said that whatever I'm doing to "keep it up!" Well, what I'm doing is a daily dose of Loving Meditations and positive affirmations. Both my doctor and I are thrilled!

~ RH from Pennsylvania

APPENDIX A—MEDITATIONS AND MINDFUL MINUTES

Meditations on the *Loving Meditations* app:

To download the app, go to CalmCancerStress.com

iOS App Tutorial

This short video will help you get started using all the features of the *Loving Meditations* iOS app.

Calming Your Stress and Anxiety

As you enter into lush scenes of beautiful nature, you will be carried toward a deep sense of peace and calm. The breathtaking images, Tamara's soothing voice, and David's expansive music will help you feel grounded, centered, and tranquil.

Cancer2Calm—Caregiver

As a caregiver, your judgments around cancer may be impeding your journey to peace. Surrender into complete calm with this powerfully releasing meditation. (Also available in Spanish)

Cancer2Calm—Patient

As a cancer patient, your judgments around cancer may be impeding your journey to peace. Surrender into complete calm with this powerfully releasing meditation. (Also available in Spanish)

How to Meditate Successfully

Tamara shares the eight keys for a successful meditation experience to help you achieve the best results.

Quick and Easy Mindful Breathing

Experience peace and calm within minutes with this easy breathing technique.

The Gift Cancer Gave Us

David is suddenly hit with a diagnosis of stage IV cancer and Tamara puts everything on hold to be his caregiver. Even though this cancer journey had its challenges, they were able to see the gifts in this experience!

Waiting Room TV Soar

As reported on CNBC, 63 percent of surveyed patients say that the most stressful thing about going to the doctor is waiting. This excerpt from the *Loving Meditations Waiting Room TV* is designed to help you feel less stressed and more grounded.

You Are so Amazing!

Need an emotional boost or inspiring words to improve your mood? Watch this uplifting video to ease your cancer journey today.

Five-Minute Mini Vacation

This journey through the vibrant fall colors of Vermont takes you on a mindful mini vacation ... perfect for calming while in the waiting room.

Awaken. Allow. Attract.

This powerful visualization will help you pull energy from the perspective of abundance, to attract what you desire in your life.

Calm4Chemo

This meditation is meant to be watched before or during your chemotherapy, and will assist you in receiving a more positive experience.

Catch Your Breath

Take a moment to catch your breath. Feel peace and calm within minutes. Perfect while waiting for the doctor or health care services!

Chakra Clearing Meditation

The human body has major energy centers called *chakras*—spinning vortexes of energy. This meditation will help clear stuck energy from every part of your body, helping you feel centered and balanced.

Experience Blissful Sleep

A sleepy, gentle, and effective guided journey that induces deep relaxation and sleep that will last for hours.

Feel Life: All Is Well

If you are living with cancer as a survivor or caregiver, this visualization will help you put your awareness on life and living on this beautiful planet.

Gratitude: Say "Yes!" to Life

Make gratitude part of your daily practice. It can boost your mood, help you focus on the positive and put a brighter filter on your day. Follow along with this powerful guided-meditation and say "yes" to life!

Heartbeat (Release Emotions)

Body tapping is highly effective for releasing stuck or heavy energy, especially negative emotions. By tapping over your heart, you will feel more open, free, and positive within minutes.

Inhale. Exhale. Relax.

This simple yet effective meditation helps you to become hyperaware of your breathing while shifting you into a state of calm.

Judgment Detox

When you are judging yourself or others, it doesn't feel good—not to you or anyone around you. Judgment is toxic. This visualization will help you to operate from a place of greater freedom and allowance.

Loving Your Body to Sleep

Gratitude for your body and relaxing breathing carry you into a profoundly restful state in this guided journey to sleep.

Mindful Walking

David's motivating music and Tamara's upbeat directions will inspire you to get outside and move, giving your body the gift of healthy walking.

Nausea Relief Meditation

Watch this meditation to dramatically reduce nausea, dizziness, or foggy brain. By visualizing your own roots growing deep into the earth, you'll feel more balanced and grounded.

Refresh. Revitalize. Renew.

Pull in energy from around you to feel refreshed, revitalized, and renewed in minutes.

Release Pain and Discomfort

Your mind and body will take a relaxing vacation by using these powerful yet gentle breathing techniques. Before you know it, you'll reach your goal of reducing, and possibly eliminating, pain and discomfort with ease.

Releasing Your Fear

This meditation is designed to help you reduce fear and leave you with a sense of renewed calm and peace.

Mindful Minutes:

The following are quick tips to help patients and caregivers experience more ease during their illness experience.

Reset Switch – How to view our challenges as an opportunity to create something new.

Mindful Downtime – How we can use downtime in waiting rooms for positive benefit. As cancer patients and caregivers, we spend many hours waiting!

Nourishing You – Caregiver Alert! How to identify the most important thing you can do for yourself every day.

Being Present – How to focus on the present rather than on your worries.

Letting Go of Attachment – How to let go of attachment. What if caregiving a loved one provides that opportunity?

Making It A Win-Win – How to get creative when someone is asking, "What can I do to help?"

Shift Your Focus – How to shift out of mental chatter and feel more grounded.

Holiday Tips: Be Stress Free – How to release anger, especially helpful during the upcoming holiday season. Tamara shares some quick and easy tips.

Holiday Tips: Make a List – How to handle people who push your buttons during the holidays. Tamara shares a fun, practical tip.

Made in the USA
Middletown, DE
30 November 2022

16532765R00109